The Roots of Pelvic Floor Yoga

Women Releasing Shame and
Reclaiming Confidence, Freedom, and
Radiance From the Inside Out.

Heather Dolson, R.N., BScN

Although I am a nurse, I am not your nurse. The medical and health information provided in this book is for general, informational, and educational purposes only and is not a substitute for professional advice. Accordingly, before taking any actions based upon such information, I encourage you to consult with the appropriate professionals. I do not provide any kind of medical/health advice.

Thank you for choosing this book!

I created a free 3-day video series

Pelvic Freedom

to introduce you to practices that

bring awareness to the pelvic bowl and pelvic floor

and support you to regain confidence.

Go to this link and get it.

www.heatheronhealth.com/pages/pelvicfreedom

Contents

Introduction

You've heard your fitness instructors or physiotherapists going on and on about the pelvic floor and the pelvic bowl; *"you are rotating it too much," "you've tilted it too far this way or that way,"* or *"that it's tucked too far in that direction"* ... on and on they go. What do they even mean? What exactly is the pelvic bowl? Well, think of your pelvis as an actual bowl with hinges around your hip joints. Imagine that this pelvic bowl – or should we call it a *bowlvis* is filled to the brim with your favorite liquid. Maybe water, a smoothie, soup, it could even be coffee? So, what happens when you tilt this bowl forward or backward? You guessed it. The liquid will spill all over. Same if you tilt it sideways, it will spill everywhere. The bowl has to be in a neutral position if the liquid is to stay inside, which often happens when you are in your sitting and standing position. Your pelvis initiates all the movement in your spine and hip joints. The pelvic floor, therefore, contains all the important muscles and connective tissues that support your pelvis and all the organs inside it.

But why is this important, and why am I talking about this? Because I believe we have to start from the basics. Indeed, the pelvic floor is the powerhouse of the female body, but many of us know nothing about it. As a registered nurse and a yogi passionate, I have witnessed this firsthand. Whenever I ask a client to engage their pelvic floor, some will jerk their pelvis forward. Others will suck their abdominal muscles in and grab their glutes, forcing their bladder downward. This doesn't change their pelvic floor in any way. They've either tightened it too much, or it's not involved in their movement in any way. The pelvis and the pelvic floor muscles are not only helpful in preventing back pain and urinary or bowel incontinence that usually happens due to age, childbirth, pregnancy, and other neurological disorders. A robust, upright posture has its foundation in the pelvic floor. In fact, your pelvic floor muscle tones and your pelvis' general position speak volumes about how you face life in general. Moreover, the pelvic floor has been proven to be the seat of a woman's passion, lust, and pleasure, whether or not they have a partner.

Research shows that women are more vulnerable to pelvic floor dysfunction because of its direct association with pregnancy, menopause, and childbirth. These are issues that affect women. The National Institute of Health reports that an estimated 1/3 of adult women will experience some kind of pelvic floor dysfunction and its related conditions at some point in their lives. Another 30% of those women might require corrective surgery to deal with its symptoms. Think about this; half of the world's population is made up of women who have vaginas. These women have uteruses, and they give birth and raise children. Why is it that women, and society as a whole, are utterly clueless about issues surrounding the pelvis, pelvic health, the pelvic floor, and pelvic floor dysfunction? It indeed concerns me that such important issues surrounding women's health and other natural cycles are somehow taboo and are still at the very bottom of conversation lists today.

When I first thought about and sat down to write this book, I asked myself many questions. I thought about my experiences with urine leakage after the birth of my two children. I spent many hours reading about pregnancy, postpartum effects, and urinary/bowel incontinence that happens after birth. But when I was experiencing all these, I felt alone in my problems. My pelvic floor issues really came in the way of me enjoying some of life's little pleasures, including playing with my kids, exercising, and things felt different with sex! This resulted in embarrassing problems relating to urinary incontinence when my kids asked me to jump with them on the trampoline or when I would go for a run, leading to less social engagement.

And I tried to share those problems with friends, family, and doctors. Their responses were often casual, *"things change after giving birth, you know this, right?"* they would say. The truth is they didn't get it because they hadn't experienced any of this. In a way, I understood where they were coming from. Still, this didn't help. My vagina had changed, yes! But I wasn't mad about that, even though that, in itself, deserved mourning. But as many women can agree, I was heartbroken because I couldn't pee and play like I used to. I leaked urine whenever I coughed, sneezed, or laughed, and this wasn't the most challenging aspect of it. I learned that women were often shamed for these issues. Pelvic floor dysfunction comes with its embarrassing symptoms, but being shamed for it by society and not being able to speak up because these are "taboo topics" makes it ten times worse. I also learned that I wasn't alone in this. Studies show that 25% of U.S. women struggle with pelvic disorders, including urinary and fecal incontinence and pelvic organ prolapse.

For many women, the damage sustained during childbirth went deeper than the superficial vaginal tears stitched up after delivery. I realized that more happens in these cases. The connective tissues often tear off from their anchor points and are unable to function as required. I didn't know this was what had happened to me. I only had my intuition to rely on.

Writing this book was genuinely healing for me. I was embarrassed at first, and this was reflected in my first draft. But with every revision, my shame and embarassment focus on self reduced as I realized I wasn't alone in this. Many modern women carry a lot of pelvic issues that interfere with their physical, emotional, and energetic flow. I found myself imagining what it would be like for a woman in her senior years to notice that part of her cervix was now protruding from her body or a young 22-year-old mother trying to adjust to having urinary and fecal incontinence while taking care of her new baby or a 40-year-old mother of five too busy to seek medical care for her painful genitals or urine leakage even when resources are within reach. I was genuinely moved by these thoughts, as I'm sure many of you are reading this. I thought to myself, "*how about I get that ball rolling and look for ways to help such women?*" How would I do this? By using my knowledge and personal experiences to empower other women.

Indeed, women from all walks of life have been dealing with pelvic floor disorders since the beginning of time. The earliest medical records in history show that this is true, and there is a possibility that women were dealing with these issues long before then. Studies show that many women turn to surgery to fix these problems. But, there is enough evidence, following multiple studies and years of research, showing that pelvic floor muscle training and pelvic floor yoga can give an alternative method to avoid surgery. In addition to my experiences as a mother of two, I am a registered nurse and a yogi passionate; I have been for more than 18 years. I have also studied medical research literature extensively and know that pelvic floor yoga and other pelvic exercises work. It worked for me; I no longer have urine leakage issues and I have more pleasure and satisfaction with sex. I have also helped my clients overcome these issues using evidence-based alternatives to surgery. My goal is to see them happy and to help them achieve urinary continence, bowel continence, a better quality of life, confidence, and pleasurable sex.

In all my years working as a registered nurse and now as a holistic pelvic yoga instructor, I have always been incredibly curious about the female body. Why are women struggling with pelvic floor pain? Why are women dealing with so many pelvic pain conditions? Why have these issues been normalized? Why are issues surrounding women's health never discussed openly? Heck, why are women just expected to *"live with it"* – *"that's just what being a woman is all about,"* insert big rolling eyes! No! You should NOT be silent about these issues. You shouldn't be living with these problems because *"things change after birth. That's just how it is."* These issues deserve an explanation point. Ladies, these patterns need to stop.

I have always leaned toward healing and treating a person as a whole. I want to challenge healthcare professionals to slow down and listen to these stories, truly listen to their patients' stories in full. This is not about bashing any of them, as I am one myself. This is about challenging them to do more. They've always advocated for better care for women, but let's not stop there. The ball is now rolling, so it's time for the real work to begin. In this book, I share my ideas on what changes I'd like to see, but I also know that we must start by educating ourselves – all of us. We must learn to feel comfortable with having these uncomfortable conversations with women. And it may be something as simple as being silent, listening intently, and absorbing all the details of a patient's story.

Emotional connection is truly important for women going through these issues. Sitting with them and sharing in their discomfort is true care. Leaning into their vulnerability and extending a helping hand is true care. I know these gestures are powerful and empowering. This is what I give to my clients. I give them a helping hand and an emotional connection, showing genuine concern and care for their problems. This is what we should all do. Doesn't this make perfect sense, though? When someone is dealing with pain, fecal and urinary incontinence, lack of libido, an inability to enjoy sex, and the fear and anxiety about being out in public because of how they need to modify their behavior when leaving the house, don't you think that they would feel some shame and vulnerability. So, now you see how critically important (women's health, particularly pelvic health) that we, as a society, assess a situation, talk about these problems and treat the person as a whole. Our bodies deserve more care; to receive this extra care, we must first understand our bodies.

My professional life prepared me for this. I have the expertise and knowledge that helps me read into and interpret a client's physical patterns. I examine the physical structure to understand the underlying issues that stand in the way of a woman's vitality, those issues that require adjustments. Regarding the female pelvic bowl (its root), pain patterns (emotional and physical), disconnections, and congestions through assessments. I 'map' their pelvic bowl to gain insight into the cause of a client's pain and other conditions such as constipation, pelvic organ prolapse (POP), and urinary/bowel incontinence.

I have learned that the root patterns and the structure of a woman's wild feminine range can be altered and expanded. Using tools such as pelvic floor yoga, a woman can restore the vitality of her root muscles – the most powerful and critical muscles that support female bodies. Working on your roots (pelvic floor) will refine your awareness of all subtle sensations. You will begin to feel the warmth of your creative energies because yoga helps you strengthen and tone your pelvic floor. You'll recognize your power and understand how much energy your pelvic bowl holds. Through pelvic floor yoga, you'll find a real connection between your creative capacity and the state of your root.

Taking care of your pelvic floor/root is the first step toward learning to speak with your feminine voice. Start by visualizing and bringing awareness to your pelvic bowl. I will show you how you can do this successfully in the next chapters. We must honor our pelvic bowls. Both intricate and joyful associations with our pelvic bowls are valuable in restoring pelvic vitality. Every awareness in the pelvic area increases its connection with other body parts. The pain and sensation of wounding give guidance for healing. The pelvis is a powerful base for general posture and support. When you honor it, you will increase its capacity to physically, emotionally, and spiritually support you.

As I continued writing this book, I also realized that I wanted other professionals in the medical field to read it. So, this book is for you, too, if you are a pelvic floor physiotherapist, general physician, obstetrician, gynecologist, and everything in between. It's crucial for us in the medical field to understand a patient from their own perspective. This rarely happens during the limited time patients come in for appointments. Most importantly, I want to encourage women to educate and empower themselves. There's still room for improvement in women's health and related areas.

You picked this book for a reason; you could be pregnant, have just had a baby, or want to strengthen your pelvic floor muscles. It's good that you are making an effort. I am proud of you. Whatever the reason, this book will be like the lighting of the torch that gives you a comprehensive guide in your journey of strengthening your pelvic floor. This book provides the information you need by sharing strategies that you can use to combine yoga and other pelvic exercises with research-based practices so you can fully recover from pregnancy and birth. Understand that this isn't limited to pelvic floor renewal only; yoga adds so much positivity and light into your life. Yoga has many benefits, including improved mental clarity, flexibility, calmness, mindfulness, and overall well-being.

Everything you'll read in this book reinforces a cycle that, once set in motion, builds upon itself in positive ways. And the good news is that you already have all you need inside of you. You should look forward to an amazing, intuitive, and deeply moving journey – a journey into understanding your power. A journey into relearning your body's lost wisdom. No, this book contains no mindless strategies that require you to push yourself too much. Treat this book like a spa visit where you learn more about your core, and you come from it as a sensual, healed, and relaxed woman full of energy and zest for life.

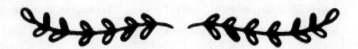

Chapter One

Pelvic Floor Dysfunction

The Effects on the Quality of Life and Mental/Emotional Health

I t is absolutely heartbreaking to see that issues surrounding women's health remain taboo among the general population, even though women make up 51% of that population. What's more, healthcare professionals have many unique opportunities to influence women's health throughout their lives positively. Many of those interactions revolve around other issues other than ill health, such as pregnancy prevention, safe sex, healthy menopause, healthy pregnancy, pregnancy loss, and life post-menopause. To be more impactful, we must promote the importance of rarely discussed issues – including those that affect women at different ages and stages of their lives.

Studies show that the 21st century has brought the biggest group of adolescents in history. Therefore, they must learn early that it's possible to take control of their physical (particularly reproductive) and mental health. For this to happen, young women and men must be educated and informed early so they are empowered enough to seek help early. As it is, pelvic floor dysfunction is a critical concern affecting a high percentage of women, especially those who've experienced childbirth and pregnancy – yet it remains a highly sensitive and taboo topic for many people.

Research highlights the prevalence of pelvic floor dysfunction in women – up to 23% will experience at least one or another kind of pelvic floor disorder at one point in their life. This probability also increases gradually with age ranging from up to 10% in women aged 20-39 and up to 50% in women aged 80 and over. Understand, also, that the probability of pelvic floor dysfunction increases significantly after pregnancy and birth. Take pelvic organ prolapse, for example; it may affect up to 50% of women who've given birth. This may happen immediately after birth or many years down the line. Up to 40% of women interviewed by the Alberta Women's Health Foundation reported pelvic floor dysfunction and other related issues, including incontinence and prolapse.

"I've had to rearrange my life around my symptoms; I've canceled many social events or physical shopping days because of it. The condition has also substantially influenced my decision to retire." - study respondent struggling with pelvic floor dysfunction.

Studies have suggested that because we've been conditioned to think of pelvic floor dysfunction as a "part of life," women often feel shamed, guilty, and stigmatized to talk about it. These conditions affect women in many ways. It negatively impacts their sexual life and, in turn, sexual relationships and restricts participation in many activities. The stigmatizing and taboo nature of the condition has pushed many women into silence, so they don't seek help as soon as possible. The Alberta study reports that 57% of women admit that pelvic floor issues have impacted their professional life in one way or another, and another 68% have agreed that it impacts their home life negatively. And even when women gather enough courage to seek help, they also have to deal with significant physical and psychological impacts brought on by delays in treatment.

Despite its prevalence, few women are even remotely aware of the possibility and likelihood that they will deal with pelvic floor issues until they actually are dealing with it and need medical attention. This is something that needs to change. That's because up to 90% of age-related incontinence cases can be improved with exercise, and 70% can be improved with physiotherapy. Tools exist. Solutions and help for women suffering from pelvic floor dysfunction do exist.

It's frustrating that the medical system doesn't support people with pelvic floor issues enough. These issues are normal; why aren't we discussing them more openly? As I said, a majority of my clients admit that they've never even heard of the pelvic floor before. No one has ever mentioned to them the need for rehabilitation after childbirth, whether vaginal or cesarean. This problem cuts across cultures, social classes, societies, and religions.

Understand that these disorders can range from mild to severe, so different women dealing with pelvic floor dysfunction could have very different experiences. For this reason, I've always felt the need to hold lunch-and-learn seminars, webinars, and conferences with other medical professionals and physiotherapists, teaching them how to draw their patients in and educate them on the importance of staying active during and after pregnancy. I've always tried my best to provide my clients with valuable information to help them recover after pregnancy and birth so they can minimize and prevent damage to their pelvic floors.

Still, I am continually surprised and even heartbroken by how little first-line healthcare professionals know or educate their clients about pelvic floor dysfunction and pelvic floor in general. They know a lot of things; that's a fact. But there is a lack of patient education and support about the pelvic floor, yet they are right at the front with pregnant and new mothers. Clinical practice and first-line treatment guidelines are clear; pelvic floor rehabilitation should come immediately after delivery. But this isn't what's made available in healthcare systems at the moment.

To add insult to injury, pelvic floor issues are extremely expensive for the healthcare system in general and for the patients, obviously. Depending on a patient's location and the type of insurance they have, physiotherapy can be hard to access, and even when it's accessible, it could cost an arm and a leg.

And surgery is an option, particularly in severe and persistent incontinence and prolapse cases. Surgery involves a mesh sling attachment designed to provide support to the urethra. The mesh sling keeps the urethra closed, preventing urine leakage even under pressure. But this isn't a permanent solution either. The effects only last about seven years. The surgery has also become controversial in recent years. Worldwide reports indicate different types of complications associated with these devices. Thousands of Canadian and American women have reported that the mesh intended to help has, in fact, eroded inside their urethra, resulting in excruciating pelvic pain and other complex autoimmune issues. Eventually, the American Food and Drug Administration stopped the sale and distribution of the said surgical mesh.

Canada quickly followed suit, banning the mesh implants used to treat pelvic organ issues from their market. This happened after a health and safety review from Health Canada. Indeed, this surgical mesh can still be used, according to Health Canada, but in very specific patient groups. This included patients with recurrent pelvic organ prolapse issues and others at a high risk of undergoing other forms of surgery.

Other women also admit that physiotherapy isn't enough to fix their problems. One study participant shared that she struggled with incontinence for over 16 months following back-to-back pregnancies. This happened even amid weekly physiotherapy appointments and other forms of treatment. She describes her experiences as "living in constant fear," always worried about knowing exactly where the bathroom is so she can rush there where necessary. This study participant hit her breaking point and decided to proceed with the surgery anyway. Now, she feels like she has her old life back. *"This is freedom. It's quite liberating,"* she says.

Links between pelvic floor dysfunction and mental health

The prevalence of pelvic floor dysfunction is much higher in women. That's because there are so many injuries associated with the pelvic floor, including but not limited to menopause, hysterectomies, obstetric trauma, the effects of diabetes, UTIs, neurological disorders, and aging, which are more common in women. Pelvic floor dysfunction becomes more common and severe with age. The increased risk has also been linked to cognitive and neurological disorders, stroke, and traumatic brain injuries. Developing nations have a large percentage of rapidly aging populations, increasing the percentage of people dealing with pelvic floor dysfunction and the resulting mental health issues.

Incontinence resulting from mental disease

Some mental health disorders, such as dementia, could make a person so confused and distracted that they never get to the bathroom on time, leading to incontinence. Moreover, certain medications used to treat mental health disorders are known to cause urge incontinence. Others reduce bladder sensations that give the brain and nervous system urination signals.

Another reason could be the ingestion of unreasonable quantities of diuretics and bladder irritants like alcohol and caffeine. Finally, certain lifestyle choices may bring about chronic ill health that affects basic bodily functions such as urination. For example, smoking can lead to persistent cough, which will, in turn, weaken the pelvic floor in the long term and cause or aggravate different forms of incontinence.

The association

Serotonin is a chemical/neurotransmitter that could explain the link between incontinence and depression. Depression can lead to more production of cortisol (stress hormone) and catecholamine (produced in response to physical/emotional stress) in the bloodstream. These two powerful hormones could lead to changes in bladder function, resulting in urinary incontinence. This means that depression and urinary incontinence may have additive effects on each other.

Incontinence as the cause of mental illness

Incontinence has been linked to increased weakness, aches, and increased risk of falling in seniors as they rush to get to the bathroom in time. Now, let's say they decide to use diapers or commodes; this will ultimately affect their sense of independence and dignity leading to depression and social anxiety. This alternative is also known to result in loneliness and isolation. I have been a nurse in long term care and the prevalence of this exact situation is heartbreaking and all too common.

Incontinence is highly embarrassing and is known to make people shy. They may avoid social contacts and social activities as well. This means that a person isn't just dealing with incontinence, but loneliness and isolation, which can lead to significant self-neglect, depression, and even death. This is particularly true in older people, so healthcare professionals must educate them on these conditions, their impact, and available treatment options.

With urinary incontinence more prevalent in women, the chances of depression are shown to be 80% higher compared to 40% higher in moderate or mild cases of incontinence. Anxiety symptoms worsen by up to 50% in women with urinary incontinence. Research also shows that the prevalence and degree of anxiety are likely to multiply four-fold in severe incontinence cases.

Fecal incontinence is even worse, with an even greater level of shame for the ordinary patient. The prevalence of anxiety in fecal incontinence patients is four-fold, and the rate of depression multiples by up to five times, together with mild/intense feelings of social ostracism, desperation, guilt, humiliation, and shame. This is particularly associated with the fear of fecal incontinence in public, where a patient may be unable to hide it.

Left in the dark

The conversation surrounding women's health continues to shift. Many women have come out to speak boldly about their experiences in the healthcare sector. These include misdiagnosis, lack of information from proper and extensive medical research on women's issues, and the struggles associated with being taken seriously by medical professionals. Many women have felt, at one point or another, that they aren't being listened to or are being brushed off. This often happens when they gather enough courage to speak about their issues. Even worse, older women, who are amongst the most vulnerable group when it comes to pelvic bowl dysfunction, report feeling "invisible" to health professionals. Women, throughout their lives, have to deal with a lack of empathy and sympathy around issues relating to pregnancy, pregnancy loss, menstruation, infertility, childbirth, incontinence, and menopause, according to a new study.

A study done on older women struggling with reproductive issues reports that they often feel "brushed off" and "invisible." Others feel like they are not being listened to like they should or that their symptoms aren't taken as seriously as they would appreciate. Many carry with them a feeling of "being in the dark" about their physical and mental health. A 45-year-old woman in the focus group opened up about her experiences, *going to the doctor isn't a fun experience because they rarely listen. That's my problem. Now, I just don't bother going.*"

Women also raised the issues surrounding support and information and how they are often difficult to find. There was a general perception of a lack of therapies, inadequate help and services, follow-ups, and support for women dealing with pelvic floor dysfunction and its related problems. The researchers noted that many women, therefore, preferred silence. This silence cut across women of all ages but was most prevalent in older women, who have many caregiving responsibilities. Research shows that women live longer and are more vulnerable to different types of disabilities later in life. Yet, older women consistently reported being "brushed off" and "written off," with many struggling to find the support they need. The research also revealed that women face many uncertainties about their health and access to relevant and helpful healthcare services.

"Invisible illnesses," as often described, are at the center of conversations about women's health. Indeed, healthcare is constantly growing, and treatments are being innovated, but reproductive, hormonal, and gynecological issues affecting women are still behind. Many women believe that these disparities are deeply rooted in the "invisibility" of their issues. What makes the situation even worse is that many hormonal and gynecological issues are extremely difficult to diagnose. Let's take endometriosis, for instance – as much as it is experienced by one in every ten women; studies show that it takes an average of 8 ½ years to diagnose. But even as the conversations surrounding "invisible illnesses" expand, women (like the older women mentioned in the previous paragraph) feel invisible too. A lot has been said about how much women suffer in silence.

Research from Endometriosis UK research shows that up to 62% of women will consistently put off visiting the doctor's office with gynecological health-related symptoms. The said 62% cuts across women aged 15-64, with many admitting their reluctance was associated with feelings of embarrassment, fears of not being taken seriously, or not thinking that their symptoms were serious enough. The statistics are much worse in 16-24-year-olds, with 80% having the same thoughts and feelings. What do these studies and statistics reveal? There's still a lot of stigma surrounding women's health, and many women still believe whatever they are going through is normal. These findings raise many questions about reproductive, gynecological, and hormonal issues. What's the price society pays for upholding these stigmas? How can these stigmas be broken down – medically, socially, and psychologically?

Some argue that the existence of "invisible illnesses" speaks a lot about our society's toxic normalization of pain. This extends to mental health issues because when you aren't okay physically, you are struggling emotionally as well. A recent inquiry on issues surrounding pain and mental health in women reveals that 90% of women dealing with any type of pain or illness would appreciate access to psychological support, but many didn't get it. When dealing with such issues, depression, anxiety, and hopelessness creeps in and is extremely common.

Mary Lee Baron, Ph.D., RN, FNP-BC, in her 2008 study, confirmed that the prevalence of mental health issues, including depression and anxiety, increased significantly following reproductive health events in women, such as puberty, pregnancy, childbirth, postpartum, perimenopause, and menopause. Mary also reported a 10-15% increase in symptoms of major depression following childbirth. Many people may find it surprising that there's still little to no medical research into these areas. After all, at least half of the population may encounter these difficulties at one point or another. The call for change, support, and public awareness for women dealing with pelvic floor dysfunction poses the question of what support and change really mean. One of the best ways to support women in such issues is to build upon existing research.

Certain conditions surrounding reproductive health are called "pain illnesses" and may be disbelieved or ignored. Some people argue that even though "pain illnesses" can severely impact an individual's quality of life, they still lack enough support and research. Add these to complex and extensive diagnosis times and minimal possibilities of treatment, creating awareness around these "invisible" and "pain illnesses" become more necessary than ever.

Beyond medicine, research reveals that acknowledgment is a critical first step in supporting chronic pain patients. Education is undoubtedly important, but pelvic floor dysfunction and related illnesses are also known to impact people differently. This also extends to friends and family who could be affected by having a loved one suffer from these illnesses. Communication then becomes important. Increased awareness and an understanding of the illness should extend not just to the person suffering but to their partners, friends, and family as well. As is the case for many women dealing with pelvic floor dysfunction, there is barely any support and information for partners. Many partners feel left out and marginalized from issues that affect them. It's uncommon for partners to share or even be asked how it feels living with patients and how this condition affects them, albeit indirectly.

Creating space for people with pelvic floor dysfunction to share their experiences without shame or embarrassment and listen intently and actively to sufferers is important in increasing awareness and empathy for those affected. Indeed, these conversations are adapting, calling us to areas that need keen attention – areas that have been skipped over or normalized in the past. Maybe the first step is to reduce stigma; as it is, the normalization of pain is the foundation of many issues affecting women's health. Even as we learn to become more inclusive as a society, it's important we look at issues felt by women globally. Improving healthcare for this section of the population is an important first step in empowering women and pushing the idea of inclusion and gender equality.

The emotional impact of taboo topics surrounding women's health

Taboo topics and shame associated with issues affecting women don't impact our emotions only. It also affects our physical and mental health. Research findings demonstrate that when a woman is ashamed or embarrassed about something, she is less likely to seek help or medical advice. This leads to late diagnoses, which may result in the worsening of the condition. The saddest thing about it is that even if you were to make it to a doctor early, you may never get the level of attention and care you need. I mentioned that women feel "brushed off." Still, even if that wasn't the case, research shows that issues affecting women are under-researched and highly under-funded – taboos and stigmas have kept them at the very bottom of conversation lists.

Ultimately, even the most well-meaning medics may be under in-formed and ill-prepared to give women the necessary help and sup-port. Again, not speaking out against certain conditions exacerbates stress and worsens existing health issues. All it takes is a little confi-dence to talk about these issues; this can be highly transformative.

One of the biggest taboos in women's reproductive health, and also a personal one to me, is incontinence. Urinary and fecal incontinence is an incredibly isolating experience and, sadly, not uncommon. Stress incontinence, for example, affects 4-14% of young women. All forms of incontinence have a certain level of psychological consequences, including shame and insecurity. In the end, stress incontinence could lead to depression, anxiety, avoidance, low self-esteem, and isolation, yet this is still a shameful subject. Why?

Society tells us that we should suffer silently. And why is that? So that if we suffer, we do so privately and quietly? At first glance, it may seem/sound like a strategy that protects our well-being, but in reality, it doesn't. It only isolates us, cutting us off from supportive networks when we need them the most. It's also unfortunate that incontinence lies at the intersection of two taboo topics – mental health and women's reproductive health. Incontinence can have long and devastating effects on a patient's mental health. But these are uncomfortable facts, and no one wants to talk about them – and they are certainly things no healthcare professional wants or is prepared enough to deal with. Many women report feeling unsure, even un-supported when seeking incontinence information. Routine mental health checkups are rarely given to women following childbirth, and general physicians who haven't specialized in women's health have proven to be ill-prepared gatekeepers. Many are unsure about talking to women about reproductive health, let alone treating them.

And it's not just pregnancy, childbirth, and pelvic floor issues that suffer the pain of being put in a box labeled "taboo." Female pleasure also falls under the same umbrella. We already know incontinence is closely associated with shame and guilt. How, then, will women enjoy sex when dealing with two of the most stigmatized topics in our society – female pleasure and incontinence? It really is a double-edged sword – whichever way you look; there's no winning. Ultimately, all these issues fall through the cracks of healthcare and are almost always forgotten.

Women's health has been sidelined for the longest time by both medicine and business – two critical areas highly dominated by our male counterparts. Do you think this is a coincidence? Absolutely not! If we can't talk about our own bodies, if discussing our bodies makes us uncomfortable, why would we expect men to do it for us? Doesn't it make sense that men also always shy from these so-called "taboo" conversations?

Women, we need to stand up for ourselves. It's time we became our own advocates and not wait around for someone to do it for us. It's pointless blaming others and pointing fingers when we can start and keep these conversations rolling. A traditional approach to healthcare hasn't served us since time immemorial. How about we demand more, create products and services we can easily access, and ensure women's needs are at their very core? How can you do this? How about not shying away from these conversations and demanding more from the system? I've asked myself this question too. How can I contribute to women's health? And then I realized I had life-changing knowledge and experience from my years working as a nurse and a yoga instructor. *"Maybe I can write a book and teach women about pelvic floor dysfunction,"* I said to myself.

I could show them another way. I could share with every woman, local and beyond, the importance of yoga – pelvic floor yoga and all its benefits in women's reproductive health. I've always been a big believer in education and awareness. Awareness is the first step towards closing the gap caused by shame. I mean, the ball is already rolling. Investors are slowly recognizing the importance of this sector – big companies are looking for and getting the financial backing they need to invest in women's health. Elvi, a brand that caters to breastfeeding and pelvic floor dysfunction, recently closed one of the biggest investment rounds - $42 million, to be exact. Clue, a popular menstruation tracker, has raised over $27 million to support issues relating to women's health. Bayer recently took over KaNDY Therapeutics, a biotech company working around menopause-related issues for over $1 billion. It is evident that people are making a real effort to break the taboos on women's health and that this is a multi-billion dollar industry.

But this isn't just limited to breaking taboos and overcoming stigma; it's about closing the care gap caused by guilt, shame, and embarrassment. This is about making everything easier for patients to connect with healthcare professionals and encouraging women to speak about issues that have been avoided in the past. This isn't limited to creating products that solve problems but building brands that spark these conversations. I am proud to be on this side of history, playing a small but significant part in ending the shame and closing the health gap by teaching women about pelvic floor dysfunction and how pelvic floor yoga can help them so that, ultimately, we can all live shame-free, happier, healthier lives.

Chapter Two

All Things Taboo

Hysteria, Wandering Wombs & Vaginas

To close the gap on shame and embarrassment and break the taboos surrounding women's invisible health problems, it's important to turn to history and the roots. This is not something new!

Yes, hysteria is a gendered insult. You'd be intrigued to learn that this started way back than we all thought – centuries ago, actually. I'll talk about that in a minute.

In 2017, the Senate intelligence committee urgently called Attorney General Jeff Sessions in. They wanted him to talk about his Russian contacts and their links to Donald Trump right before the 2016 elections. These hearings were discussed by people all over, as is always the case when it comes to anything Russia. One of these conversations led to a heated, odd exchange between then-Senator Kamala Harris and Jeff Sessions. An analysis of the conversation between Harris and Sessions included an intense argument between Jason Miller–

Trump's advisor at the time, and Kristen Powers, a journalist and political analyst. In that conversation, Miller claimed that Jeff Sessions had done a good job at pushing off Harris's "hysteria." The exchange between Miller and Powers lasted for a few good minutes. Most of it was Powers disagreeing with Miller, arguing that we should all get a pause before we describe someone as "hysterical." Eventually, an analysis of this analysis resulted in several claims supporting the idea that calling Senator Kamala Harris "hysterical" was, in fact, a gendered insult.

That's right – it happens even to the most accomplished and powerful of the lot.

Many women can testify to being called hysterical, particularly in personal and professional relationships. I've actually experienced this in a relationship when I expressed emotion; I was called "hysterical" or "irrational." So, one has to question; where do these subjective misconceptions come from? Why is a show of emotion, especially from a woman, hysterical and misunderstood?

You'd find it fascinating to discover that the word "hysteria" is used in relation to female words 49% of the time. If you compare that with only 14% of the time it is used in relation to male words and 23% in mixed groups, you can't help but wonder – why? How did we come to this point? I'll tell you this – the origins of the word "hysteria" have something to do with this. And the idea of hysteria didn't end with women's voting rights either. The American Psychological Association approved the use of "hysterical neurosis" as a diagnosis up until late 1980. That's just a few decades ago, and we still wonder why shame still exists for women and issues surrounding women's reproductive and mental health. Women have been shamed since time immemorial and that's why many prefer silence.

If I were to ask you to imagine someone crying hysterically, you'd most likely picture a woman losing it; a woman who's out of control, right? Why? Well, it's not your mistake – this isn't some personal failing, at least not entirely. It's proof we've been conditioned to associate "hysteria" and being "hysterical" with women.

Let me explain *hysteria*

We now think of hysteria as irrational panic, but it wasn't always like this. At first, the word was used to describe anything "characterized or relating to hysteria." For a long time, hysteria was, in fact, a medical diagnosis. The Greeks argued that when a woman behaved irrationally – or in a way they would consider irrational- it was because her uterus was wandering around her body, giving her trouble. The Greeks also linked different types of attitudes and "ailments," (in women) including anxiety, nervousness, irritability, boldness, sexual desire, outspokenness, and confidence to hysteria. The origins of the word hysteria have strong links and ties to the idea that any expression of emotion from a woman is proof of her inherent fragility and instability. The echoes of these same ideas are still present in our society today.

The Greek word for suffering in the womb, "hysterikos," is where the phrase "hysteria" comes from. It was stigmatized as a taboo topic in women's health since it was thought to be a medical issue historically connected to women. In the nineteenth century, female hysteria was a medical condition frequently identified in women and thought to be brought on by uterine problems. It was assumed that the groundwork for diagnosis was a sex-related interpretation of differences in stress responses, which held that women were prone to mental and behavioral problems. This idea was not supported by facts but by myths and superstitions.

In the modern medical world, doctors doing medicine no longer accept hysteria as a medical diagnosis. It has been fragmented into numerous categories, e.g., epilepsy, dissociative disorders, histrionic personality disorder, or other medical conditions. Additionally, lifestyle choices, e.g., choosing not to marry, are not considered symptoms of hysteria.

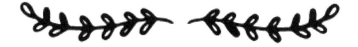

History of hysteria

The history of hysteria goes back centuries. It can be traced back to ancient times when it was thought that the uterus was a living thing that could move about the body and wreak havoc on a woman's health. The theory of the wandering womb was the name given to this notion. Undeniably, hysteria is the first mental ailment attributed to women, as it was narrated in the second Millenium BC until Freud reviewed it as a female-only disease. For about 4000 years, this disease was seen from two angles: scientific and demonological, linked to witchcraft and demonic possession.

Women who exhibited symptoms of hysteria were often accused of being witches and were subjected to various forms of torture. It was thought that hysteria could be brought about by a series of bad habits, including reading novels (that caused sexual fantasies), bisexual behaviors, masturbating, and homosexual behaviors. These resulted in some symptoms, e.g., irrationality, seductive behaviors, functional paralysis, general troublemaking, and contractures. There were also a couple of cures: for those who viewed it as the result of witchcraft, sex, and herbs, recommended sexual abstinence, punishment, and purification through fire, and those who clinically studied it as a disease recommended treatment through innovative therapies. There were also many pages of misleading medical information whereby "treatment" was administered through genital massage from an approved provider, intercourse, and marriage. Some new methods were introduced, including ovariectomies and cauterization of the clitoris. Hysteria was first documented in about 1900 BCE in Egypt.

Ancient Egypt

The Eber Papyrus, the earliest known medical text that mentions depressive symptoms, dates back to 1600 BC. It contains descriptions of a condition that was thought to be similar to hysteria. Suffocation of the womb is a condition mentioned in the Ebers Papyrus and is characterized by symptoms like abdominal pain, breathing difficulties, and a sense of suffocation. The ailment was apparently brought on by the uterus shifting and pressing against other organs. In ancient Egyptian culture, there was a belief that the cause of any illness, whether physical or emotional, was brought about by an imbalance in the body fluids, humors, that is, blood, phlegm, black bile, and yellow bile. Even if one was out of balance, a disease would attack.

Hysteria is also often associated with the goddess of beauty, love, and fertility, known as Hathor. It was believed that women who upset her would get infected. The first recorded case of hysteria in Egypt, dates back to 1900 BC, where a woman started showing the symptoms.

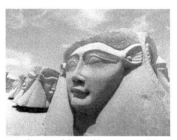

Hathor, goddess of beauty and love

Initially, they categorized hysteria as a physical disorder characterized by convulsions and paralysis. It was also believed that emotional disturbances, such as stress and anxiety, could cause it. Hysteria became a common ailment in Egypt through the centuries. A philosopher and physician known as Avicenna, wrote widely about hysteria during the Islamic golden age, describing it as a disease caused by excess black bile.

Ancient Greece

In Greek medicine, hysteria was believed to be a uterus disorder. Hippocrates, the Greek physician, also called the father of modern medicine, was among the earliest to describe hysteria in medical terms. He was the first to use the word hysteria. In his literary works, he describes it as a condition whereby the uterus is filled with blood and causes symptoms like anxiety. He also comprehensively defined hysteria and how it differs from epilepsy. He stresses the distinction between hysteria, brought on by the unusual movements of the uterus in the body, and the compulsive actions of epilepsy, which are brought on by a brain condition.

He believed that the treatment for hysteria was supposed to focus on restoring balance to the body, and he recommended treatments like exercise, massage, and aromatherapy. Hippocrates also believed the disease was more common in women and linked to the menstrual cycle. Hysteria became a topic of discussion among Greek medical scholars. Thereby, other Greek physicians, such as Galen, studied the condition. Galen believed hysteria resulted from a lack of sexual activity and recommended sexual intercourse and marriage to treat and prevent it.

Despite having medical significance, hysteria was used in social and cultural situations. It was often used to explain the behavior of emotionally volatile women. It was also used to reinforce gender roles. The relation between hysteria and women continued to be a focus of medical discourse throughout history.

Ancient Rome

Ancient Romans rejected the conventional notion of a wandering uterus and instead linked hysteria to an anomaly in the womb. They believed that hysteria was caused by a womb ailment or a problem with reproduction, like a miscarriage.

Galen, a Greek who followed up after Hippocrates, was now a Roman physician. He was one of the prominent figures in the development of hysteria-related medical theory during this time. Galen held that when one of the four internal fluids known as the humors—which were supposed to control health in ancient medicine—were out of balance and that this was what produced hysteria as reported by Egyptian medicine. He specifically thought that excess black bile, which he connected to the reproductive system, was what produced hysteria. Galen shared Hippocrates' view that hysteria was more prevalent in women than men and influenced by the menstrual cycle. To address the problem, he suggested therapies, including massage, aromatherapy, and exercise.

Hysteria in ancient Rome had cultural, social significance, and medical relevance. Women thought to be experiencing hysteria were frequently viewed as a threat to societal order and occasionally faced social stigmatization and legal repercussions. This was especially true where women were believed to be using their hysteric symptoms to attract sympathy or attention from others.

Only Soranus, a Greek physician who practiced in Alexandria and Rome and is credited with founding scientific gynecology and obstetrics revolutionized hysterical treatments. According to Soranus, women's disorders are caused by the strains of reproduction, sexual abstinence is the key to recovery, and perpetual virginity is the ideal state for women. Fumigations, compressions, and cataplasms are ineffectual. The hysterical body should be treated with care: exercise, hot baths, and massages are the best prevention of such women's diseases.

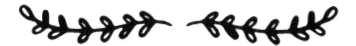

Hysteria and mental health

Hysteria has been used as a common name to describe a range of symptoms, mainly in connection to mental health conditions. Over time, hysteria has been linked to various medical and psychological needs as its concept evolved. The conditions involved are mood disorder, personality disorder, and anxiety disorder.

Throughout history, hysteria was used to describe a condition thought to be exclusive to women. To summarize, the disorder was believed to come from the female reproductive system. The treatment was administered through interventions like removing the uterus and massages. As time passed and people got a better understanding of mental health, it became evident that the disorder of the reproductive system does not solely cause hysteria.

Hysteria is considered a manifestation of anxiety and stress in modern psychology. Hysteria displays a variety of physical as well as emotional symptoms. These include seizures, paralysis, depression, and anxiety. These symptoms are frequently shown in individuals who have experienced trauma or a large amount of stress. The symptoms are therefore an attempt by the body and mind to cope with stress.

There are multiple theories to explain the connection between hysteria and mental health. One is conversion disorder. It is caused by psychological stress, which is converted to physical symptoms. The symptoms include paralysis, blindness, or seizures that don't have a clear medical cause.

A different theory suggests that hysteria may be a form of dissociative disorder. According to this theory, hysteria is a condition where the individual experiences disconnection between their thoughts, experiences, and feelings. Its symptoms may include loss of memory and a sense of detachment, which is also a way of coping with mental trauma. Hysteria could be a manifestation of this dissociation.

Lastly, mood disorders, depression, and anxiety are linked with hysteria. A depressed person, for instance, experiences physical symptoms, which include headaches, fatigue, and muscle pain, while people with anxiety experience trembling, heart palpitations, and sweating—all of the listed result from the manifestation of an individual's emotional distress.

Hysteria might have negative connotations due to its historical association with women and reproductive health. As its concept has evolved, today, it is understood to be a manifestation of stress, trauma, and anxiety. It is a valuable concept in modern psychology that helps us better understand how our bodies and minds respond to stress and trauma.

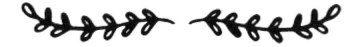

The wandering womb

The issue surrounding women's reproductive health has been tinted with devaluing women. The theory of the wandering uterus is one example. They believed women to be the weaker sex because of menstruation and pregnancy, both psychologically and physically. By the late nineteenth century, it had been scientifically established that women's anatomy rendered them less rational than males and unsuitable for participation in many facets of public life. Many people believed that women's pain and sicknesses were brought about by the wandering uterus. According to Hippocrates and other physicians, the uterus was like an animal moving around the body hungry for semen.

The wandering womb in ancient medicine was believed to cause suffocation and death. The Greek physicians suggested that hysteria resulted from a nomadic uterus. According to them, the uterus could detach itself from its original location and move about the body, causing many health issues for women. For instance, the uterus might shift to the gut, resulting in digestive problems, or move to the heart, resulting in chest pains. In return, this would make women hysterical. No one had an idea on how to prevent this from happening, but one cure that the physicians were sure of was anchoring the uterus, and this could easily be achieved by either impregnating the woman (believed that the fetus would anchor the uterus to its proper place) or keeping the uterus moist through sex. Sex would make sure the uterus does not detach itself in search of moisture from other organs in the body.

The result of the womb's nomadic nature was to create emotional and physical turmoil until the uterus found comfort. As a consequence of this, the women had fainting episodes, menstrual cramps, and verbal inconsistencies. Hippocratic physicians prescribed some treatments that included vagina fumigation (placing a sweet smell around the vagina and foul salt by your nose to lure the uterus back to the women's groin. Aretaeus suggested that the uterus was attracted to or repulsed by a particular smell, causing either prolapse or hysterical suffocation. If the vulva was drawn to a smell, it would distend out of the vagina towards it; if it was repulsed, it would ascend toward other organs. Thus, smell could be used to realign the uterus. Other treatments included bitter portions, balms, and pessaries made of wool by the skilled masseuse.

Doctor S.Weir Mitchel, one of the practitioners who gained popularity in the 19th century as a hysteria physician, championed what he called "the rest cure,". It allowed sick women to be put to bed, instructed not to move around, asked to do creative work of their liking, and drink milk every two hours. These types of treatments were prescribed to famous women like Virginia Woolf and Edith Warton. Greek doctors also recommended animal waste (cow, goat, or bird waste) in combination with sweet-scented wine or rose oil as treatment. Remedies derived from animal waste are still employed in modern medicine; for instance, a form of estrogen used in post-menopausal hormone therapy is produced from pregnant mares' urine.

Even though wombs are no longer shifting in strange places, the medical industry continues to categorize the deformities of women's reproductive system, from discharge to menopause.

Shame and taboos associated with the vagina and vulva

Women's bodies, including their vaginas, used to be worshiped as the embodiment of anatomical design. Women were valued in their roles of giving life and of earth protectors. At some point, we held at least, if not the same superior position as men. Almost all cultures have a maternal goddess who honors the cycle of life. Where did we go wrong? When did we start body-shaming women? When did we start setting the standard of how women's bodies should look?

At the beginning of this century, male professors claimed that studying Greek or mathematics would damage women's wombs. The vagina shaming goes back to when people were not exposed to information about female anatomy. When Greek Hippocrates believed the uterus was like an animal within an animal causing women sickness, they also believed that the wandering womb was attracted to the pleasant smell.

Taboos around women's genitalia are holding them back, giving women loads of insecurities. We have long been fed with information that our bodies are something to be ashamed of and should be hidden, and it's taboo to talk about any of it. This information is more triggering when it touches our intimate areas, especially our vaginas.

However, society and culture somehow propagate such taboos and exploitation of women's bodies. This makes many women uncomfortable with their genitalia. Others are also ignorant of and ashamed of themselves. Our culture has long and consistently concealed, shamed, or sexualized women's bodies, creating a hostile environment for typical, healthy representations of and relationships with ourselves. One of the biggest battles we have to fight as women is that of our bodies, particularly the vagina and vulva.

Many women are self-conscious about the looks of their vulvas and vaginas. Most women have wondered whether their labia are too long, short, fleshy, dark, light, or wrinkled. However, just because something doesn't appear perfect to you doesn't necessarily indicate something is wrong. It's important to keep in mind that vaginas and vulvas come in a variety of sizes and shapes.

ANATOMY OF THE FEMALE EXTERNAL GENITALIA

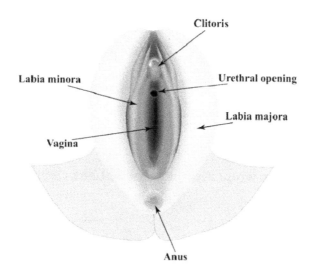

According to a survey carried out by Refinery29 (Gil, 2019), almost half (48%) of the 3670 respondents were concerned about the look of their vulva or the outside part of their genitalia (including the clitoris, labia minora, and labia majora). 64% were most frequently concerned with their size and form (60%) and were almost as concerned with the color of their vulva (30%). These worries coincide with the rising popularity of labiaplasty, which increased by 45% globally between 2014 and 2015, and the new trend of vaginal bleaching. Does this mean that someone is simply creating insecurities and then taking advantage of them? This could be true because, from all angles, women are fed myths that there is a way the vulva should look.

A lot needs to be done so we can have a world free from the shame surrounding our vaginas. Many of us are uncomfortable about our private parts, and most ladies don't look at them or touch them. The internet is scary and has made many women insecure about their private parts by comparing theirs with what is uploaded. Most of us don't understand that they may seem 100% symmetrical, but the owner has had several labiaplasties to make them look the way they do. It is becoming a trend to have bikini wax or Brazilian waxes. A few years ago, women did not even shave their legs, leave alone their pubic hair, and now most women are doing it, making the rest who don't ashamed of their pubic hair and start thinking of how ugly they are.

Why are women embarrassed about their vaginas?

The term vagina should be normalized, and no shame should be associated with it. Women learn to be ashamed of their body parts from the reaction of those around them. We were taught to cover up and not touch ourselves as kids. Our body parts were given nicknames such as "down there" or "private parts" instead of proper terms. As a mother with a daughter, I do not shame her when she touches herself. This is normal and curious exploration. I do, however, tell my daughter "those are your lips or labia." Women often feel embarrassed to talk openly about their vaginal problems and many remain uninformed. Due to a lack of information or shame, we deal with complicated issues in the long run.

Here are some reasons why women are ashamed of their vaginas;

- **Feminine hygiene**

Feminine hygiene is a multi-billion dollar industry that invests in giving women access to sanitary products and convincing them that the

scent of their vaginas is unattractive. Internal cleansers, such as the
douche and intimate spray, are the fastest-growing product category in
the market despite doctors' advice against using them. Labiaplasties,
or operations to change the vulva's look, are also rapidly increasing.
There was an 80% rise in the number of young women who un-
derwent the procedure between 2014 and 2015. Most of the language on packaging products for vaginal hygiene, such as gels, sprays,
deodorants, wipes, and douches, implies that the vagina should be
odorless, hairless, and discreet. Since at least the 1930s, when scents
were added to menstrual pads to cover up natural odors, this myth has
been propagated. But that doesn't inherently imply that the additives
are safe.

- **The porn industry**

The media creates most of the naked women you see, and any "hanging
out" parts have been altered to create perfect images. In the porn business, women appear weaker by being made to resemble young girls. If
you compared yourself to someone, you would definitely end up with
self-esteem issues. We are not little girls; we are lovely, mature adults.
It's not shocking that seeing a surgically altered, perfectly lit, waxed,
or bleached vagina in motion can make women feel insecure about
themselves. Who even noticed that their vulvas appeared any different
from the next girl's when a big bush was in? The current trend of fully
or mostly shaven privates exposes all our "flaws" in public. However,
they are all remnants of the idea that women's enjoyment should
be a subject of condemnation and shame. This has led to increased
labiaplasty as women want to change their vulvas to look like what
they saw.

- **Not knowing what is normal**

Women do not seek answers when something seems wrong, and we question whether what we are going through is abnormal. The search for the ideal vagina may never end due to a lack of knowledge and open discussion about what is perfect concerning the look and function of female genitalia.

Some women may be tempted to undergo procedures like labiaplasty and the O-shot to correct flaws they "hate" or think are abnormal. And it's probably from media sources like women's magazines that feature airbrushed, unrealistic genitalia that they get the notion to despise their bodies. These pictures might foster viewers' insecurities or expectations of what's "normal," which would explain the rise in vaginal rejuvenation procedures.

• Partners

Vagina shaming does not end with girlhood, and many men quickly reinforce those feelings throughout a woman's adulthood. Sexual partners could make you uncomfortable and question how you look down there if they negatively criticize your vagina. This can include criticizing the size, shape, or appearance of the vagina, as well as expressing disgust or disinterest in engaging in sexual activities involving the vagina. Most men's views on female body appearance are mostly skewed by porn, and with this, they have made women feel like their vaginas are abnormal for not matching porn standards; others would comment on the color and mention that it is not the same as what they saw. It is important to note that your partner is fortunate enough to be anywhere near your vagina.

• Giving birth

The vagina changes naturally after birth: it could get stretchy, loose, and even tear. Tearing during birth is normal, especially if the child is big. The tear leaves a scar, and because we have been brought up to think our vagina should look some way, most women do not embrace the scar, but instead, they become more insecure about their appearance down there. They lose their confidence, and some won't let their partners go down on them to receive oral sex.

- **Vagina smell/odor**

Our vaginas and vulvas have been through a lot, and each one is unique, whether in shape, color, or how they smell. Every vagina comes with its smell and taste, as influenced by several things. For example, our drinking water habits, what we eat, and even our periods impact the vaginal odor. There is no specific vagina smell; the vagina is home to bacteria and comes with its Ph. If you notice a fishy smell, that should be an awakening call to visit a gynecologist.

Things you need to do to fall in love with your vagina and vulva

Only after we learn to appreciate our vulvas will we be able to develop a healthy measure of self-confidence. But given the long-standing negativity surrounding vulva and vaginas, that is a difficult thing to do. It is said that many of us today can't correctly name our anatomy. Many of us only understand that our worth is measured by appearance, size, and color, even our vaginas. Learning to love your vulva will also help you love hidden things. Women with no confidence in their vaginas have low sexual satisfaction and self-esteem.

- **Study the female anatomy**

Many women cannot correctly identify the parts of the female anatomy, so don't worry; you are not alone. Take responsibility to better understand the parts of your genitalia and to locate them, even if it takes you looking at your vagina in a mirror. Know what changes and looks like when you are turned on. Do gynecological visits to learn basic vaginal education.

- **Look at other vulvas**

The media frequently distorts women's bodies, and vulvas are no exception. The distinction is that we hardly ever see real women's vulvae. Our only depiction is typically through mainstream pornography; try searching for an amateur focusing on natural bodies. According to research, many women are unaware of what a "normal" vulva appears like, and a huge percentage haven't seen one since watching those misrepresented sex-related video tapes. You'll be able to accept your vulva more easily if you realize that vulvas appear in various shapes, forms, and colors. No matter their shape, color, or pubic hair style; exposing yourself to a range of vulvas can help you see yours as beautiful and individual.

- **Be surrounded by "Vagina Love"**

Developing a favorable body image can occasionally be simpler with a little external motivation. Start simply. In your own home, watch and consume media that promotes sexual self-esteem. You can count on your gynecologist to create a friendly environment where vulvovaginal knowledge is shared, and inquiries are welcomed. Demand respect and a passion for providing you with pleasure from your intimate companions. Attend unique local shows like The Vagina Monologues or other events.

- **Understand what's normal and what is not**

It is normal for women to discharge occasionally, so it's crucial to know what that looks like for you so you can recognize changes in your fluid balance. Understanding what to anticipate can help you take charge of your fertility, whether trying to get pregnant or purposefully avoiding motherhood. Cervical fluid has different consistencies at different points in your cycle. Birth control pills, medications, sexual exercise, and diet can all alter the consistency of this fluid.

- **Pick a good partner**

Find a spouse who compliments you on your vagina and expresses their appreciation for it. They must never make negative, judgmental, or demeaning remarks about your genital area. Giving constructive criticism—such as, "I'd turn on you if you trimmed your bush" or, "I'd adore it if you took a shower when you got back from the gym before I went down on you"—is one thing. It is quite another thing to humiliate you, refuses to lower yourself, or otherwise cause you to feel self-conscious or uneasy about this area of your body.

Remember that even though you're still working on your present situation, your wonderful partner who wants to give you oral pleasure is undoubtedly attracted to your lady parts. Don't take away his or her enjoyment. It's worthwhile to overcome your self-criticism to fully appreciate this act and establish a close connection with your partner and yourself.

- **Masturbation/Self Pleasure**

Another taboo topic is one of the things most of us do but will never talk about it. The fact that we are ashamed to talk about it only means that most women don't get the benefits they should from masturbation. It is a pleasurable activity that helps you better understand and appreciate your vagina. Knowing what turns you on, on your own can help improve confidence during sex. How can you know or tell someone else what you like, if you do not know?

- **Love your labia**

They appear in various shapes and sizes, but they are all normal despite these variations. We've established some aesthetic norms that specify the type of genitalia that is desirable, but this shouldn't be a justification for you to suffer with your labia.

Unless it is a problem for you, the easiest way to learn about your labia is to study it, examine it closely in a mirror, and touch it. Do it frequently to keep track of any form or color changes and even to keep an eye out for lesions and new moles. Embracing your vagina and vulva is very important to embrace your sexuality, womanhood, and yourself.

Chapter Three

Sexuality, Pleasure & Orgasms

F rom public forums in the Roman Republic to modern internet forums, women have experienced judgment and ridicule because of their perceived sexual conduct throughout history. Women are often reprimanded for actions, clothing, or desires that are seen as more sexual than society considers appropriate. Personally, in my own expression of boldness and sensuality in the online space, I have also received derogatory comments such as "freak," "slut," and "whore" and have been requested not to post sensual Boudoir photos as this was being labeled as "pornography."

Slut-shaming is a topic that brings to light the social problems brought on by the double standard. This is because slut-shaming typically targets women rather than men. Due to its high-context society and ease of victim blaming, slut-shaming is pervasive in our society as a whole.

Here is some evidence of slut shaming in the past and present:

The Republic of Rome

Ancient Rome may have birthed the slut shaming stereotypes associated with the dress code that we see today. Women's sexual desires were categorized based on their dress code. Married women could be differentiated from sluts by how they dressed. According to Lewis Webb - virtuous women were meant to wear the stola, and prostitutes wore a toga or other symbols of trade. Married women struggled to be sexually virtuous and were punished for being overly sexual. We cannot ascertain how slut shaming made women feel or respond to it; there is no evidence written by women that refers to such occurrences. Still, we know that the origins of slut shaming run deep and will be here for a long time.

Shakespeare

In his popular comedy "*Much Ado About Nothing*," a woman is horrendously slut-shamed by her father and fiancé due to untrustworthy rumors about how she conducted herself sexually.

World War 2

After World War 2, gender roles were redefined, and so was sexuality. The theme of sexual education films revolved around female sexuality and how it threatened male dominance. Men's roles during the Second

World War were mainly breadwinners. While women were socialized and instructed to embrace the cult of domesticity and homemaking, men constituted most of the labor force.

According to author Emily Poole, the sexual revolution of the 1960s and 1970s led to an increase in premarital sex and the use of birth control. And in the 1960s and 1970s, feminist authors like Betty Friedan, Gloria Steinem, and Kate Millet inspired women to be open about their sexuality, even in public places.

The Internet Era

In the era of the internet, slut shaming is becoming popular. Slut-shaming is widespread on social media sites, especially the most popular ones: Facebook, Twitter, Instagram, and YouTube. On Facebook, slut-shaming has taken place in contentious discussions between users that have led to convictions for threatening, harassing, and causing offense, and women are the targets. Slut shaming is gender-based; When it comes to sexuality and expression, females are denied the freedom enjoyed by their male counterparts. Women are judged by society when their behaviors are made public.

Internet users who have been subjected to slut-shaming can occasionally speak out about their experiences, critique popular media, and join in on debates that were previously taboo. Other times, the internet gives people a platform to use nasty language to develop into incredibly menacing harassment, violent threats, and actual violence.

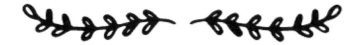

Sexual Shame and Sexual Health

Sexual shame refers to a feeling of disgrace or disgust towards one's own identity as a sexual being. It's not a secret that there is a lot of judgment when it comes to sex; that is why there are fewer and fewer talks about sex. It can be difficult to avoid these judgments or feel free about your sexual desires. Sexuality is almost always associated with shame and the core of feeling flawed and unacceptable, leading to a feeling of unworthiness and, therefore, unloved.

The biblical story of Adam and Eve illustrates the beginning of sexual shame. After sinning, we are told Adam and Eve covered their private parts with fig leaves after realizing they were naked. The fig tree represents the beginning of shame in sexuality, desire, and our traditions. We are hard-wired to cover our sexuality by wearing "appropriate clothes," secrecy around sex, and giving little to no information on sexual education. We cannot openly discuss sex and sexual desires with others.

Sexual health is a vital aspect of overall health and well-being, yet many women struggle with sexual dysfunctions; female sexual disorder refers to a variety of issues that impact a woman's ability to engage and enjoy sexual activity, including low libido, difficulty achieving an orgasm and pain during sex.

Female orgasmic disorder refers to the inability to experience orgasms even after being sexually stimulated and aroused. At the height of sexual excitation, people have orgasms which are profoundly delightful feelings of release and uncontrollable pelvic floor contraction. Even after sufficient sexual stimulation, many women still struggle to experience orgasms with a partner. Both psychological and physiological issues can cause female orgasmic disorder. A female orgasmic disorder diagnosis may cause personal distress or problems in a relationship.

Negative impacts of sexual shaming on sexual pleasures and functioning

Sexual shaming refers to a situation where someone is made to feel ashamed, guilty, or humiliated of their sexual preferences, behaviors, or wants. It can take many forms, including societal norms, family values, media representation, and educational practices. It can also take the form of cultural and religious beliefs. Sexual shaming can negatively affect a person's sexual functioning and pleasure in a variety of ways, including:

Sexual shaming can result in a distorted and negative self-image. When someone feels inadequate or inferior due to their sexual impulses or habits, it can undermine their confidence and lead to low self-esteem. They may find it difficult to express themselves, explain their wants, or fully enjoy their sexual experiences as a result.

Lack of communication and closeness in partnerships can result from sexual shaming. When someone feels shamed for their sexual demands or habits, they could find it awkward or embarrassing to express them to their partner. This may cause misunderstandings, arguments, or sexual dissatisfaction, which can obstruct intimacy and connection.

Disgust. This is brought about by carrying around shame and being judged or you judging yourself. You should explore your body; having sexual challenges does not mean you are disgusting.

Sexual shaming can cause sexual fear and anxiety. Someone may feel guilty or uneasy about having sex if they are criticized for their sexual desires or actions. As a result, one may postpone having sex, have less desire for sex, or have trouble achieving sexual arousal or orgasm.

Inhibited desire and arousal. Shame is like a thick coat that blocks a natural, healthy sexual desire and arousal response. Shame hinders you from enjoying sex.

How to embrace sex without shame

Women dominated by sexual guilt and shame tend to hide their sexual behaviors or desires because they see them as undesirable or unacceptable. A person's ability to connect with others is hindered, and isolation develops through hiding and concealment. However, to embrace sex, you need to tackle and overcome your shame. Shame can put up barriers in your way of having satisfying sexual experiences. To completely embrace and appreciate your sexuality, it's necessary to resolve any shame or negative thoughts about sex.

Ways to overcome your shame;

- **Educate yourself**

Gaining knowledge about sexuality, sexual health, and pleasure can aid in understanding and accepting your sexual needs. Finding information, busting stereotypes, and eradicating preconceptions about sex can be eased by resources like books, podcasts, and online platforms.

- **Challenge the messages that are trapping you and identify where they are coming from**

Having a method to express your thoughts and emotions can be a terrific place to start and an option for processing problems later. Writing them down is the most effective way to achieve this. Putting these thoughts down on paper could enable you to explore further and identify the source of your feelings. In the future, how do you hope to feel and view sex? And how can you healthily pursue those objectives? Write all these things down and start working on them.

- **Establish what makes you feel better when experiencing a shame spiral or feeling down**

Do you need to solve problems? Do you desire connection and empathy? Or do you wish to be diverted? Find out what might help you overcome feelings of shame, and then do more of it. This can sometimes include naming it, sitting in silence until the feeling passes, and engaging in an enjoyable activity. Other times, the best strategy is to locate a distraction or another person to chat with until you feel like you can handle things again.

- **Communicate with your partner**

You could feel prepared to talk about your thoughts with someone you trust once you feel more at ease expressing your emotions. This could be discussing sex in general or expressing some of the thoughts and feelings you've recorded in your journal about sex. If you want to communicate with your partner, learning what you like and dislike can help. Having open lines of communication with your partner can make you feel at ease and secure during sexual encounters. Discuss your boundaries, desires, and preferences to ensure you and your mate are on the same page.

- **Consult a professional**

Think about getting help from a therapist or counselor who focuses on sexual health and wellness if you are having issues with sex-related shame or guilt. Sexual shame and guilt can be deeply embedded issues, even though there are certain initiatives you can take on your own and with the support of loved ones. They can provide strategies to deal with your emotions and help you accept your sexuality without feeling ashamed.

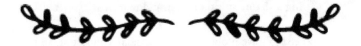

Advertising shapes women's ideas of sex

Advertisements frequently use imagery to elicit emotions, moods, and ways of being. However, sex is frequently portrayed in advertising in an idealized or exaggerated way that does not reflect actual experiences. A good example of this is lifestyle branding, which involves showcasing the idea behind sex through an image or set of images that conjure up a desired and plausible world that a person is urged to see themselves existing and engaging in. Advertisements may present sex as always passionate, spontaneous, and ideal, leading to unrealistic expectations or poor perceptions of one's sexual encounters.

Although the constructed setting mostly depicts the ideal rather than reality, it is presented to the viewer in a way that makes it appear reachable. This is evident in magazine advertisements depicting how sex is constructed in society. In addition to the information, the American idea of sex is also for sale. Advertising can employ lifestyle branding to impact how society views sex and sexuality and to persuade women to pursue the ideal sexual state rather than to accept and enjoy the actual sexual experiences they have in their lives. For example, they may perpetuate negative gender roles or stereotypes that restrict women's sexual agency or encourage negative attitudes toward sex. Instead of portraying women as active and empowered sexual beings, advertisements may show them as passive and submissive or as objects of male desire.

Advertisements also reflect how sex and sexuality are viewed in American culture. Advertising is a potent informational tool and cultural relator. Advertising is a type of cultural text that sheds light on the society in which it exists and serves as a reliable indicator of the level of sexual tolerance in an era. On one level, magazine advertising is acceptable to society, while on another, it reflects the sexual attitudes of society. The meaning we perceive from commercials is based on commonly held societal assumptions, perceptions, and values, which advertisements influence to convey a particular meaning to the viewer. Ads that convey society's perception of sex through visual means construct their pictures on that conception while also going beyond it.

When women view sexualized advertisements, they try their best to identify with the feminine aspects of the ads and apply the messages to their lives. Unrealistic standards and ideas are further normalized by the widespread adoption of overly sexualized representations of women. Advertising does this by extracting meaning from a certain context and then re-creating or representing it. Since none of us are living up to the ideal, it is vital to redefine oneself when attempting to relate to an ideal image of sex, sexuality, and sexiness. No matter how unrealistic they may be, women often strive for the ideals and ambitions presented in commercials. Thus, to conform to the female descriptions in advertising, we modify our bodies, refigure how we look, and redefine our sexuality. Because the representations are continuously shifting and unreliable, the issue is that we never succeed.

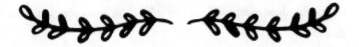

Disconnection between women and their own sexuality

Despite major strides in gender equality, women still encounter significant obstacles in accepting their sexuality. Women have been conditioned to regard sex as shameful or unclean practice, which should be kept private and avoided amidst conversation. Because of this, women no longer feel connected to their bodies and are reluctant to dig into their wants and desires.

There are many reasons for this disconnection, they include;

- The way sex has been portrayed in popular culture is one of the main causes of this divide. Instead of being active participants in their sexual experiences, women are frequently portrayed as passive objects of male desire. This downgrades women by supporting the stereotypical ideology that sex is something that men do to women rather than a choice women make for themselves, and further, that you should be embarrassed about your urges.

- The commodification and objectification of women's bodies

in the media is another aspect that contributes to this divide. Women's sexual needs and wants frequently take a back-seat to their physical attractiveness, from airbrushed images in fashion magazines to hypersexualized music videos. This brings the feeling of insecurity and incompletion to women since they are continuously reminded that they have to look a certain way to be attractive.

- The gap between women and their sexuality is also largely caused by the absence of extensive sexual education. Many young women have little to no awareness of their bodies or sexual health as they grow up, which can cause confusion, humiliation, and even physical discomfort when having sex. The myths and biases about sex that are perpetuated by this lack of understanding include the notion that women should not enjoy sex or that they are somehow "dirty" for having sexual impulses.

- Women may experience guilt or shame about their sexuality due to societal standards on gender roles. Women are fre-quently expected to care for and nurture others; if they don't fulfill these expectations, they face harsh judgment. Due to the fear of facing society's harsh judgment, women may find it hard to investigate their urges and wants because they are compelled to believe it is selfish and not what is expected of them.

For women to fully accept themselves, they must invest their time in exploring their sexuality. Exploring sexuality can be done by; getting to know their bodies and learning about pleasure and sexual health. Creating early awareness among the youth through campaigning for proper sex education and opposing harmful gender stereotypes and social standards. There is no appropriate method to embrace one's sexuality; it is a personal journey. We can build a more welcoming and powerful society that celebrates women's sexuality in all manifestations by removing the obstacles that have historically kept women from truly engaging with their bodies and desires. Next, I will discuss how the roots of yoga weave into sexuality.

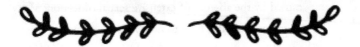

Kundalini and Tantra practices

Tantra yoga is derived from the worship of the Hindu deities Shakti (dynamic, creative, feminine) and Shiva, who stands for the dynamic and static principles of the cosmos (static, destructive, masculine). Tantra yoga practitioners try to understand how these ideas interact constantly. Tantra is a branch of yoga that merges various practices, including initiation, mudras (hand positions), visualization, mantra meditation (Sanskrit sound), and pranayama (breathing), to investigate the inner universe through the human body. It specializes in the restoration of spiritual health as well as spiritual regeneration.

The main aim of Kundalini yoga is to awaken an individual's strong consciousness or psychic consciousness so they can see a wider reality inside themselves. With the help of kriyas, breathing techniques, and meditation, Kundalini Yoga particularly aims to activate Kundalini energy. In Kundalini Yoga, the lower chakras, the first and second chakras linked to the pelvic area and sexual energy, are given focus.

Practitioners can strengthen their connection to their bodies and improve their sexual health and pleasure by concentrating on these areas.

Tantra yoga

While the word tantra has been utilized in various yogic writings over time, its context-specific meaning has evolved. Tantra originally meant "weaving or loom," but it has since come to mean "technique, mechanism, or procedure." The Kmik-tantra text provides a more up-to-date and pertinent definition: It is referred to as a tantra because it elaborates (tan) numerous, profound concepts, particularly those related to the fundamental truths (tattvas) and revered mantras and because it offers liberation (tra).

Tantra recognizes the importance of the body as a tool to explore and delight in, as opposed to expanding and directing one's awareness externally. In the past, yoga practices emphasized giving up the physical body and making a conscious effort to separate from the pain experienced in the body. On the other hand, tantra found the importance of being aware of and enjoying the body's internal energy world.

Given that hatha yoga developed from this system of yoga and that tantra offers a context for the many practices and techniques of contemporary yoga, it is crucial to comprehend the techniques and objectives of tantra yoga. Spirit and bodies of energy are cultivated in tantra yoga to build a link to connect the worldly to the divine. The cleansing, cultivation, and activation of prana and the kundalini are the main focuses of energy development. The mudra, asanas, pranayama, and shatkarma techniques use the physical body to awaken energy. Therefore, the tantra yogis created the yoga asanas (postures) and pranayama (breathing techniques) employed most frequently in Hatha Yoga today. Hand movements and an intense combination of asana, pranayama, and bandha are included in mudras. Esoteric exercises and practices known as shatkarma (sometimes spelled kriya) purify the body and clear the energy pathways. Sanskrit sounds, known as *mantras*, are considered to be expressions of divine power. *Yantras* are sacred geometric shapes utilized in Tantric rituals to help with concentration and imagination. *Puja* is performing ritualistic offerings of food, incense, light, water, and precious stones to a deity of one's choice.

Tantra yoga was taught to Westerners in the nineteenth century as an exotic sexual and spiritual practice to increase closeness. Tantra's status as a yoga technique for amazing sex was further popularized and entrenched by the interest in Eastern spirituality and the sexual upheavals of the late 1960s and early 1970s. Tantra has historical connections to tantric teachings on the subtle energy body and the embodied presence of a sexual union. But, it is a perversion of this complex and nuanced enlightenment method to oversimplify and combine tantra yoga with sexual practices and interpersonal connection.

The Tantra Yogis' emphasis on individual exploration and experience gave rise to the radical body and mind purification methods that helped us untie the knots holding us to this world's physical reality. Tantra yoga includes a wide variety of practices, but at its core, it is about using the body as a temple to revere the sacredness of life's all-pervasive oneness. Tantra gives the practitioner a direct connection to the divine and a sense of the universe's unity. Tantra presents various yogic methods to induce ecstasy, representing a vast synthesis of spiritual wisdom.

Kundalini yoga

"Kundalini" is obtained from the Sanskrit word *"**kundal**,"* which means "circular." It is also used to mean a coiled snake. Despite being practiced worldwide, there is no known place where Kundalini yoga originated. The idea of Kundalini energy has been around for a long time and is documented in ancient Vedic texts from 1,000 B.C. Yogi Bhajan popularized Kundalini yoga in 1968. He stated that the goal of his teaching is to live a "healthy, joyful, holy" lifestyle. He showed his American students how to awaken their inner spiritual force with mantra chanting, breath practice, and yoga postures. Many Westerners looking for a new viewpoint on spirituality, wellness, and health immediately became fans of this practice and way of life.

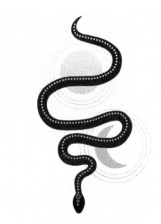

Kundalini energy like a "coiled snake"

According to practitioners, Kundalini energy is like a coiling snake; it lies dormant and unaroused at the base of your spine. Kundalini energy, or shakti, is meant to be awakened by Kundalini yoga. It can also be awakened through sexual experiences. This energy is believed to improve consciousness and aid in overcoming your ego. Kundalini yoga incorporates singing, chanting, pose repetition and breathing exercises. By awakening this energy, Kundalini yoga enables it to ascend and pass through the chakras along your spine. The seven energy centers in your body are called chakras in Kundalini yoga. The root, sacral, navel, heart, throat, third eye, and crown chakras are among them. Between the anus and genitals, beneath the root chakra, is where the Kundalini energy is kept. Tantra and Hatha yoga approaches can help you awaken this energy, which normally lies dormant and still. It then moves upward from the base after being activated. It travels via the seven chakras and the susumna, the main energy channel in the center of the spine until it reaches the crown chakra, where it connects with divine consciousness.

Kundalini's awakening results in the highest level of joy. However, unleashing this coiled snake energy might be disastrous if not done properly. In rare instances, discharging such a potent source of pranic energy into the body's delicate systems might result in mental instability and pain. Hatha yoga poses must be performed correctly to prepare the body and mind for Kundalini activation and release upwards. As Kundalini flows through the body and the nervous system adjusts to this dramatically increased psychic energy, one may suffer negative effects during an activation. As a result, it is not recommended to awaken Kundalini without the direction of a knowledgeable teacher and the backing of a spiritual community.

If done correctly, Kundalini yoga has numerous positive effects on the body and mind. This practice's intensity fosters endurance, grit, and inner fortitude. It can improve your flexibility, strength, endurance, balance, and coordination, just like other types of yoga. It eases tension and anxiety while enhancing coordination and balance. Your spiritual practice can be deepened by doing Kundalini yoga, which can aid in letting go of old patterns and behaviors.

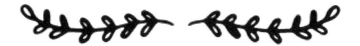

Yoga and women's sexual functioning

Female sexual dysfunction is common and often does not get the clinical attention needed. Yoga is used as a substitute and complimentary in developed countries. Yoga protagonists and patients claim that yoga is useful in treating sexual disorders and improving sexual functions.

Have you ever wondered why people who practice yoga regularly seem so happy and at peace? It could be couples who do yoga frequently experience a huge boost in the overall quality of their sex lives and energy levels. Did you know your emotional and sexual health could significantly impact your physical health? Additionally, did you know that yoga can help you feel special by focusing on your emotional reactions to life? The truth is that many students discover, as a result of attending regular yoga lessons, that their love lives are improved, their physical flexibility rises, and their taste for life becomes something to rejoice in. Why? No matter your age or how much additional weight you may have when you start, yoga puts balance firmly in your hands, and the feel-good element you acquire from practicing it regularly makes you feel alive.

Yoga helps build strength, muscle control, endurance, flexibility, and stamina in areas of the body, including the groin, abdomen, and back.

It also helps improve self-awareness, self-confidence, and sensitivity. Yoga can also help in getting better orgasms. Regular practice of child, eagle, legs up the wall, lotus, bridge, sitting wide-legged straddle, downward dog, goddess, and plow poses will improve your sex life.

Yoga relaxes both body and mind. This is one of the most beneficial things about yoga, especially for women. Yoga reduces stress that keeps sexual arousal at bay, and for women to enjoy sex, they have to get out of their heads into the sense of touch of their bodies. Female sexual arousal is found in the hormone balance and, most importantly, in the level of their stress level balance. When stress reduces, it opens the door to sexual desires and thoughts.

Yoga increases the score for sexual desires, orgasms, lubrication, arousal, and overall sexual satisfaction. Almost two-thirds of the women who practice yoga claim to be more satisfied with their sexual lives, with huge improvements in arousal and lubrication in women over age 45. You can get more control and awareness of your body by moving your body in a variety of yoga poses in a basic, slow, and controlled manner. Understanding your wants better and how you physically feel can help you communicate with your spouse more effectively. The sexual experience can also be improved by increased consciousness and a stronger sensation of being in the moment. Enhancing bodily awareness can help you stay in charge of your body better, understand your wants, and stay present, all of which can make sex more enjoyable for women. Knowing your needs before conveying them to a partner is the first stage, and yoga may support this self-awareness and mindfulness.

Yoga is used as a tool to prepare for the movement of Kundalini energy. In doing so, one may gain awareness of oneself and release the energy sustaining the source of blockage or stagnation. Kundalini energy has been said to extend the longevity of sex and elevate sexual pleasure by enabling male orgasms without ejaculation (Francoeur, 1992). Another yogic notion known as moola bandha is extremely helpful for improving sexual response in women by teaching them how to manage their bodies. Bandhas are a way to "lock," "bind," or "tie together, close" specific parts of the torso to accelerate yoga's cleansing procedures.(Desikachar, 1999, p. 71). Yoga appears to be an effective method of refining all domains of sexual functions in women, and I can personally attest to it!

Chapter Four

Welcome to the Pelvic Bowl

A Brief Anatomy Lesson

There's so much more to the pelvis than most of us think. First, we have the bones and the muscles attached to those bones. Then there are pelvic floor muscles and the deep stability muscles passing through the pelvic area. Then there are organs in and around the pelvic area. This means there is so much to feel and a lot more to think about.

We all have six pelvic bones at the time of birth; a pair of ischium bones, a pair of ilium bones, and two sides of the pubis. The two pubic bones are connected by thick connective tissues called pubis synthesis. As we grow older, these six bones fuse to form what is known as the pelvis. The pelvis is sometimes called the pelvic bowl or pelvic girdle. This bony pelvis is part of the appendicular skeletal system. It is then attached to the axial skeletal system through the sacrum. The axial skeletal system includes organs such as the ribs, spine, sternum, and skull. The sacrum comprises five fused bones just below the lumbar spine and over the coccyx, also known as the tailbone.

The pelvic floor is muscular and dome-shaped. It separates the perineal region below from the pelvic cavity above. This cavity houses the pelvic viscera – uterus in females, intestines, and bladder. A physiotherapist would therefore describe the pelvic floor as the bottommost area of the pelvis, all the structures around it, and their associated contents.

You'd be intrigued to learn that the female sacrum is shorter and broader than the male one. Not only that, but the female pelvic bones are also larger and broader than the male pelvic bones. The female pelvic bone is also lower than the male pelvic bone. The male pelvis is taller and has a raised iliac crest. This explains women's lower center of gravity, their ability to support and grow life, and the instability associated with their sacroiliac joints. This lower position of the pelvis also explains why during yoga, one would have difficulties lifting their pelvis over their shoulders, especially when doing inversions and arm balances.

The pelvis, also known as the pelvic bowl/ring/girdle is made up of the following:

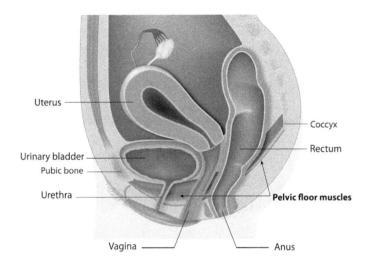

- The pelvic joint;

- Different organs, including the rectum, uterus, bladder, and their associated structures.

- The external genitalia.

- Pelvic floor musculature.

- The ligaments.

- The nerves, including blood vessels and the lymphatic system.

- Connective tissues.

- Endopelvic fascia.

Let's talk about the pelvic cavity. The pelvic and abdominal cavities are surrounded by the following:

- Abdominal wall, which creates the front border.

- The respiratory diaphragm, which creates the top border.

- The spinal column, which creates the back border

- Pelvic floor muscles, which form the bottom border

The pelvic bones

- **The hip bones**

We have two hip bones, one on either side of our bodies – the left and the right. Together, these two create the pelvic girdle. The hip bones are joined to the upper part of the skeleton at the sacrum through attachments. Each hip bone is comprised of three little bones that join during adolescence:

- The pubis: the two bones on each side connect at the joint known as pubis symphysis

- Ilium: the ilium is broad and fan-shaped and makes for the biggest portion of the hip bone. If you place your hands on your hips, you will feel the arches of the ilium.

- The ischium: your weight rests on the ischium whenever you sit down. For this reason, the ischium bones are also known as the sit bones.

Together, these three bones create the acetabulum – where the head of the femur is attached.

- **The sacrum**

The sacrum connects to the lower end of the vertebrae. It is made of five different vertebrae attached together. The sacrum supports our body weight and is quite thick.

- **Coccyx**

It is also known as the tailbone. Several ligaments connect it to the bottom of the sacrum. It comprises four vertebrae joined together to create a triangular-like shape.

The Pelvic Girdle

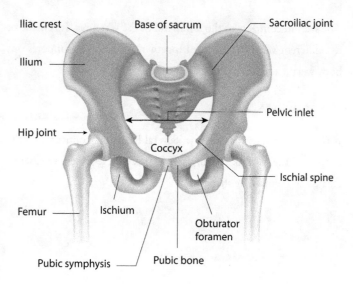

Iliac crest

Ilium

Hip joint

Femur

Ischium

Pubic symphysis

Base of sacrum

Coccyx

Pubic bone

Sacroiliac joint

Pelvic inlet

Ischial spine

Obturator foramen

The muscles/pelvic floor musculature

The pelvic floor muscles are classified into three different layers.

- **The deep layer** (also known as the pelvic diaphragm) is a broad, funnel-shaped muscle.

The pelvic diaphragm has its own muscles:

- **Coccygeus/ ischococcygeus muscle**

This relatively small muscle originates from the ischium and attaches to the coccyx and sacrum.

- **Levator ani muscles**

This is the largest muscle group in the pelvis area. It has multiple functions and helps support the pelvic organs. It has three sets of muscles;

Puborectalis. This is the muscle that holds urine and feces. When you urinate, it relaxes. It also relaxes when you have bowel movements.

Pubococcygeus. A large percentage of the levator ani muscles comprises the pubococcygeus. Coming from the pubis bone, it connects directly to the coccyx.

Iliococcygeus. This muscle has thin fibers and lifts the anal canal and the pelvic floor.

These muscles are considered more of hip rotators than part of the pelvic diaphragm.

- **The middle layer** is also known as the urogenital diaphragm

Some people also call it the perineal membrane. This middle layer contains the vaginal and urethral sphincters. These two groups of sphincters help maintain continence by closing the vagina and urethra. This middle layer also provides deeper and extra support to all pelvic floor structures.

- **The superficial layer**

The superficial layer contains the bulbocavernosus and ischiocavernosus muscles that help with clitoral function during sex and arousal.

It also has the superficial transverse perineal muscles that give the urogenital diaphragm the extra support it needs.

You'll also get the external anal sphincter within the superficial layer, a layered muscle responsible for closing off the anal canal.

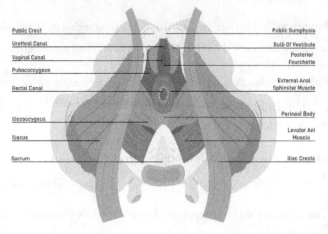

Female Pelvic Floor Muscles

Public Crest
Urethral Canal
Vaginal Canal
Pubococcygeus
Rectal Canal

Iliococcygeus
Iliacus

Sacrum

Public Sumphysis
Bulb Of Vestibule
Posterior Fourchette

External Anal Sphinster Muscle

Perineal Body
Levator Ani Muscle

Iliac Crests

The organs

- **Uterus**

This is where babies develop during pregnancy. It is a hollow, thick-walled organ that sheds monthly during your reproductive years if you aren't pregnant.

- **Ovaries**

You have two ovaries, one located on each side of the uterus. These ovaries release eggs and hormones like estrogen.

- **Fallopian tubes**

These tubes connect the egg-producing ovaries to the uterus. They have specialized, hair-like structures (cilia) that help push the eggs released by the ovaries toward the uterus.

- **Cervix**

The vagina is connected to the uterus via the cervix. It can widen and allow sperm to travel through the uterus. Moreover, the cervix produces thick mucus that helps prevent bacteria from getting into the uterine wall and the uterus.

- **Vagina**

The exterior female genitalia is connected to the cervix through the vagina. It is sometimes called the birth canal because the baby passes through it during birth.

- **Rectum**

The rectum is the lower end of the large intestine. Feces stay here as they await removal through the anus.

- **Bladder**

It collects and stores urine before it is expelled. The urine travels through pipes known as ureters connected to the kidneys.

- **Urethra**

The collected urine must then exit the body somehow. Once collected in the bladder, the urine travels out of the body through tubes known as the urethra. The male urethra is much longer than the female urethra.

The ligaments

The female pelvis has broad and short ligaments.

The broad ligaments

They support the ovaries, uterus, as well as fallopian tubes. The broad ligaments extend to both ends of the pelvic wall. These ligaments are then divided into three components, attached to different areas of a woman's reproductive organs.

- The mesometrium ligaments support your uterus.

- The mesovarium ligaments support the ovaries.

- The mesosalpinx ligaments support the fallopian tubes.

Uterine ligaments

They provide the uterus with extra support. They are classified into:

- The round ligaments.

- The uterosacral ligaments.

- The pubocervical ligaments.

- The cardinal ligaments.

Ovarian ligaments

These ligaments give ovaries the support they need. They are classified into two different categories; ovarian ligaments and suspensory ligaments.

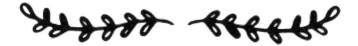

Pelvic floor physiology

The pelvic floor muscles resemble other muscles in terms of structure and function. They:

- Relax and contract

- Can shorten and lengthen

- Can be strengthened or weakened

- Can be either supple or stiff

- They can move dynamically where necessary

- They can hold tension when appropriate

- They can have or lack coordination – either as a group of muscles or individually

- They could be regulated or dysregulated normally

The pelvic floor muscles have slow-twitch fibers and fast-twitch fibers. 70% of the pelvic floor is made up of slow-twitch fibers. With so many slow-twitch fibers, the pelvic muscles can stay in a state of resting activation for a while. For this reason, they are also seen as postural muscles. The resting activation state is important because it helps maintain continence.

When necessary, the fast-twitch muscles will react, allowing for voluntary contractions, such as in the case of expected/unexpected changes in intra-abdominal pressure.

The functions of the pelvic floor

The pelvic floor has many functions, including:

- Urination

- Defecation

- Urinary and fecal continence/ sphincter function

- Sexuality and pleasure

- Parturition/childbirth

- Keeping all the pelvic organs mentioned above in the right place.

- Supporting the pelvic and abdominal viscera/stability function

- Provides extra support to the baby during childbirth

- Support internal organs and hold them in the right positions

Therefore, the pelvic floor needs a robust anatomical structure of connective tissues, muscles, and nerves to function optimally. Moreover, the pelvic floor function is also controlled by the central nervous system. This means that pelvic floor dysfunction and incontinence can, in fact, be impaired by dysfunctional neural control too. The dysfunction isn't just limited to direct anatomical injuries resulting from pregnancy and vaginal delivery. It may occur as a result of conditions related to neurological diseases, cognitive illnesses, and diabetic neuropathy.

Still, the most prevalent female pelvic floor disorders manifest as urinary incontinence (absent/decreased bladder control), fecal incontinence (decreased/absent bowel control), and pelvic organ prolapse (POP) (when the uterus, vagina, and bowel protrude from the vagina). The statistics on these disorders are a bit concerning also. Studies show that 30-50% of women suffer from one or another form of pelvic floor dysfunction, depending on which definition you use. But that's not all. The most surprising thing about these numbers is that, as high as they may be, they still don't represent the actual numbers on the ground. A large percentage of women are still not seeking care and help for pelvic floor dysfunction. These statistics support the need for more intervention and screening of patients for pelvic floor dysfunction, particularly in older women.

Women who struggle with pelvic floor dysfunction (PFD) often harbor feelings of shame and embarrassment. Many aren't honest about having these issues and would rather not share them with their caregivers. But we must understand pelvic floor dysfunction is common, and there's no need to feel bad about it. A recent Robert Koch Institute study shows that a large percentage of the population also harbors myths, prejudices, and misconceptions about pelvic floor dysfunction. This has shown to stand in the way of necessary and important prevention and care initiatives. Many people take it that incontinence is an inevitable part of aging and that treatments are not only unnecessary but also more likely to fail.

I've seen so many patients in their homes, hospital and long term care after years of struggle with pelvic floor dysfunction; many have normalized it, arguing that it results from the effects of pregnancy and childbirth and the inevitable aging. I've met young patients in their mid-20s and older ones in their 90s who arrive at the office after giving up and letting their quality of life suffer. Many only act after the effects of pelvic floor dysfunction have spilled over to other areas of their lives. You have options; you only need to ask. You shouldn't let it go that far.

Introduction to common dysfunctions and why they cause so many issues

Some sources may describe pelvic floor disorders as urogynecologic/urogynecological disorders, which describe any pain and dysfunction in the rectum, bladder, vagina, uterus, and cervix areas. These disorders are pretty common, seeing as studies report that one in every three women will experience some kind of PFD in her lifetime. The National Institute of Health reports that pelvic floor disorders affect at least 10% of women aged 20-39, 27% of women aged 40-59, 37% of those in the age bracket 60-79, and around 50% of women in their 80s and beyond.

There are no easy ways to talk about issues relating to the nether regions. Still, we have to talk about it. Pelvic floor dysfunction and other related disorders are already underreported as it is. Indeed, this is a difficult conversation because many women feel isolated in their experiences. Studies show only 17% of women struggling with urine incontinence will seek medical assistance. We already know that these dysfunctions affect more women, and of that number, 46% will suffer in silence for around 1-5 years. A whopping 42% will live with their symptoms for five years and beyond. This will obviously impact their quality of life negatively – social lives, personal relationships, and professional and other work-related activities. Pelvic floor dysfunction is also linked to social isolation, anxiety, and depression.

Please understand that there are many pelvic floor disorders, and many are often lumped together. Still, it's possible to classify them into the following subcategories; pelvic floor support (prolapse, descending perineal syndrome) and constrictor function (urinary and fecal incontinence). Furthermore, these disorders may be divided into dysfunctions of pelvic floor contraction (fecal and urinary incontinence) and relaxation (constipation and urinary retention).

It's sad that many women still believe that these are normal conditions they have to manage and live with, especially after childbirth. It's heartbreaking that many don't and won't report the sufferings they experience having to deal with the dysfunctions described below:

Pelvic organ prolapse

Some organs, such as the bladder, uterus, and rectum, are positioned around and above the vaginal canal. When the supportive tissues around the pelvic area weaken, these organs may stick out and herniate into the vaginal canal. This is medically described as a prolapse.

When it happens, you may feel discomfort and heaviness around the vagina. This may be followed by difficulties in using the toilet and unwelcome urine leakages, also known as urinary incontinence. When the prolapse is on the extreme end, these tissues may hang outside the vagina, which would make them visible. Pelvic organ prolapse manifests in different forms:

- **Uterine prolapse**

The uterus falls into the vaginal canal.

- **Cystocele**

The vaginal front wall drops, making the bladder sag.

- **Rectocele, also known as enterocele.**

The vaginal back wall sags forward, pushing the intestines and rectum into the vagina. When this happens, the rectum and intestines may be seen bulging from the vagina.

- **Vaginal vault prolapse**

This may happen following a hysterectomy. The vaginal walls may drop in such cases.

Risk factors for pelvic organ prolapse

- **Aging/menopause**

Studies show a 21.1% increased risk of developing pelvic organ prolapse during menopause. An analysis of the relationship between age and pelvic floor disorder shows a direct and positive relationship. In fact, this risk increases dramatically with each passing decade. This can be explained by the menopause/age-related hormonal fluctuations, which alter a woman's urogenital structural function. Muscle mass also decreases as we age, and this can weaken the pelvic floor.

- **The nature of pregnancy and childbirth**

The pudendal nerve may overstretch or become damaged during virginal birth. This may also happen during prolonged labor, instrumental delivery, and episiotomy (surgery done to increase the vaginal opening). The number of children and weight are also directly linked to a 4-6% increased pelvic floor dysfunction risk. Evidence from biochemical models of the pelvic floor supports these findings.

- **Genetics**

You may inherit this condition if your family has a positive history of pelvic organ prolapse. The risk of pelvic organ prolapse increases by up to 1.4 times in genetically predisposed groups. This increased risk applies when other factors like vaginal deliveries and hysterectomies aren't considered.

There is also enough proof that the connective tissues of the pelvic floor muscles may be genetically weak in women experiencing urinary incontinence.

- **Injuries to the levator ani**

This may happen during vaginal delivery or when you fall on your groin and pull a muscle. The levator ani could shift its position, and the genital hiatus may widen when this happens. When this happens, the pelvic structures will have to count on the connective tissues for support. Over time, these biological changes may cause weakening and tearing of the tissues, resulting in pelvic organ prolapse.

- **Low socio-economic status**

This is a critical factor, especially among racial minorities. Low social-economic status may lead to inadequate access to information and care related to pelvic floor dysfunction. With a lack of information, it's harder to recognize symptoms and the importance of seeking medical help as soon as possible.

When given an incontinence quiz, women of a lower socio-economic status scored lower than those of a higher socio-economic status.

Ultimately, public education to improve awareness is necessary to reduce the negative impact of pelvic floor dysfunction.

- **Hysterectomy (surgical removal of the womb/uterus)**

Hysterectomy might weaken and damage pelvic muscle, increasing a woman's risk for pelvic organ prolapse. This procedure is directly linked to multiple postoperative complications, fecal and urinary incontinence included. The same studies show a 60% increased risk of post-hysterectomy urinary incontinence in middle-aged women.

- **Previous trauma around the pelvic regions, such as falls during pelvic radiotherapy**

Pelvic radiation increases the risk of urinary incontinence in women. It also increases the chances that a woman develops pelvic floor dysfunction. Women should ask for further screening and optimal care to minimize the risks.

- **Increase in abdominal pressure**

Chronic coughing and endless sneezing, which may be signs of bigger problems, increase women's pelvic organ prolapse risks. Excessive coughing and sneezing lead to pelvic floor muscle and ligament overuse. This overuse may weaken the muscles and the surrounding anatomical structures, leading to pelvic organ prolapse.

- **Heavy lifting and constipation**

Constipation is caused and aggravated by changes in the working of the pelvic floor muscles. When the condition persists, it may lead to nerve damage and other symptoms of pelvic floor dysfunction. Jobs that rely on constant heavy lifting add unnecessary pressure to the bladder and may lead to incontinence.

Research shows that women who engaged in frequent heavy lifting were 9.6 times more likely to develop pelvic organ prolapse than the general population.

- **Prolonged participation in vigorous physical activities**

Professional athletes, particularly those who do high-impact sports like gymnastics and trampolining, often experience increased abdominal pressure from overstretching and overworking the pelvic floor muscles. Studies show that this constant strain can increase the risk of urinary incontinence.

When non-athletic women were compared with athletic ones, the findings revealed that the athletic group was 2.5 times more likely to report urinary incontinence than non-athletic women.

- **Obesity**

Obesity, as highlighted in an individual's BMI, is strongly linked to urinary incontinence in women. The urinary incontinence risk increases by up to 20-70% with every 5-unit increase in BMI. The extra weight increases intra-abdominal pressure, causing more vesical compressions and urethral movements. As the pelvic floor muscles weaken, the nerve and the surrounding structures are also affected, which leads to reduced functional efficiency.

- **Lower back pain**

Chronic back pain is closely linked to pelvic floor muscle dysfunction. The pelvic muscles provide urinary continence and stability for the lower back. But the discomfort associated with lower back pain makes people weary of any form of movement, including those that engage the pelvic floor. Disuse leads to muscle weakening and this leads to changes in urinary function. What's more, lower back pain greatly limits most people's ability to contract the pelvic floor muscles. And lower back pain is also linked to reduced motor control, leading to genito-urinary dysfunctions.

Urinary incontinence

Urinary incontinence is a widespread problem affecting millions of men and women worldwide. It can interfere with your ability to participate in normal day-to-day and other social activities. It is described as the reduction in or loss of bladder control, resulting in urine leakages. Urinary incontinence comes in many forms, so you must get the correct diagnosis before starting treatment.

There are two major types of chronic urinary incontinence:

- **Stress incontinence**

This is the most prevalent type of bladder control issue in women. It often happens after childbirth. The urine leakage may occur when you cough, sneeze, laugh or engage in exercises and other activities that exert pressure on the abdominal cavity. It could also happen in the simplest situations, such as standing or jogging.

Stress incontinence may also happen after pelvic surgery or menopause. It occurs when either the pelvic floor or urethra muscles weaken.

How does this happen? Strong pelvic muscles are important because they help hold the organs around the vaginal canal in place. But these muscles may weaken for different reasons, and when that happens, the continence mechanism around the urethra may not work as efficiently. This may result in increased abdominal pressure, which may cause urine leakage.

- **Urge incontinence**

This type of incontinence happens when you feel a strong, urgent need to urinate. The urge is so strong you can't delay it, but however much you rush, you never seem to reach the toilet before you leak. Your bladder can either squeeze or spasm during this urgency, and you lose urine before you get to the bathroom.

- **Mixed incontinence**

As the name suggests, mixed incontinence is a combination of the two bladder incontinences described above; urine and urge incontinence.

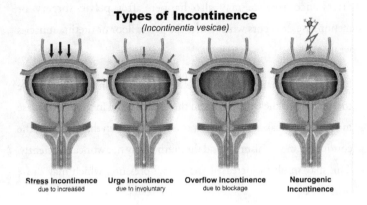

Types of Incontinence
(Incontinentia vesicae)

| Stress Incontinence | Urge Incontinence | Overflow Incontinence | Neurogenic |
| due to increased | due to involuntary | due to blockage | Incontinence |

Causes

- **Obstruction of the bladder**

This describes a blockage that interferes with urine outflow from the bladder. It may result from strictures causing narrowing of the urethra and nervous system dysfunction, particularly those associated with urinary sphincter function. An excellent example of this is multiple sclerosis.

- **Reduced contractility**

The bladder may lose its natural contractile abilities so that it doesn't squeeze out urine as efficiently as it used to. Loss of contractility may result from lower back surgeries, major bowel surgeries, pelvic surgeries, and diseases of the nervous system that are linked to bladder function, such as multiple sclerosis and diabetes.

Risk factors

Loss of bladder control is a critical, yet common problem. Still, many women don't seek care when they need to. For this reason, it is quite impossible to know the exact number of women who struggle with urinary incontinence daily.

Studies show that adult women are twice as likely to suffer from unintended urine loss as their male equals due to problems associated with the following:

- Biological differences in the pelvic anatomy's general structure

- Changes resulting from pregnancy and childbirth

- Changes related to reduced estrogen levels during and after menopause

There's not a specific cause linked to female urinary incontinence, but experts believe certain things increase the risks that a woman may suffer from it.

They include:

- Pregnancy and childbirth.

- UTIs.

- Menopause.

- Increase in weight.

- Aging.

- Hysterectomy or pelvic surgeries.

- Neurological diseases including stroke, diabetes, and multiple sclerosis.

- Pelvic radiation.

- Congenitally weak connective tissues.

- Genetics – it can be hereditary.

Fecal incontinence

Some sources refer to it as anal/bowel incontinence. Recent studies show that it is also prevalent, particularly in older adults, and is often characterized by the loss of or inability to control bowel movements. When it happens, people with the disorder may struggle to hold their stool until they get to the toilet. This may result in stool leakages from the rectum.

More than 5.5 million Americans, both men and women live with it daily. Fecal incontinence is, in fact, the second most common pelvic floor disorder. The good news is that fecal incontinence can be treated successfully and shouldn't be normalized as something that occurs with age.

It's also common for people with pelvic floor disorders to report other issues like:

- Constipation.

- Painful bowel movement or straining when passing stool.

- Urinary complications such as painful urination or inability to completely empty their bladder when urinating.

- Pelvic spasms.

- Pain around the vagina.

- Pain and pressure around the rectum.

Symptoms of pelvic floor dysfunction in women

- Numbness/pain during sex

- Chronic pain in the rectum, genital and pelvic regions

- Unwanted urine leakages

- Never making it to the bathroom in time

- Feeling of urgency in using the bathroom

- Frequent urge to urinate

- Difficulties emptying the bladder and bowel; you may start and stop multiple times

- Discontinuous urination

- Desire to have multiple bowel movements in a short time

- Bowel stains

- Constipation

- Passing wind accidentally

- Lower back pain that can't be explained by other causes

Chapter Five

Getting Started with Pelvic Floor Yoga

Yoga means union, and it is much more than physical exercise. It connects and unifies the mind, body, and spirit. Yoga is a traditional Eastern discipline that combines physical posture (asanas) with breathing exercises (pranayama). There is also a cognitive component focusing on meditation and concentration, which aids in achieving the goal of union between the self and the spiritual. Regular yoga practices come with more mindfulness, mental clarity, and self-awareness.

Yoga and chronic illness

It has recently been discovered that yoga can effectively improve our health in many ways. Whether you have neuropathic pain, diabetes, arthritis, Crohn's disease, or even Lupus, yoga can be quite helpful.

Yoga can be used as a form of treatment because it combines breath work, meditation, and physical posture that helps you gain better balance of your mind and body.

Yoga is a diverse form of therapy that makes it practical for people suffering from chronic diseases because no matter your physical limitation, there is a type of yoga suitable for you. The practice of yoga has been proven to help reduce pain, anxiety, and fatigue in chronic disease patients. Yoga postures are not supposed to be overwhelming; everyone should do what they are comfortable with. The goal is to bring calmness and happiness and release tension in the body. Yoga also activates and awakens the parasympathetic nervous system-part of the nervous system, which allows the body to rest and heal, and raises gamma-aminobutyric acid levels, a neurotransmitter that slows down your brain.

Yoga poses for chronic disease

Different yoga poses work for different illnesses; for example, corpse pose, and easy pose helps people with asthma, mountain pose and seated forward bend help with arthritis, downward dog pose and frog pose help with diabetes, and other poses like child pose and bridge pose helps with depression.

Effects of yoga

The female pelvic floor is complex and is made up of a vital set of muscles that aid in sexual, bowel, and bladder function and support the organs in the pelvis. A person's pelvic floor must be strong to be healthy and powerful. However, the pelvic floor muscles can weaken due to some causes, including aging, giving birth, and inactivity. These can cause health problems, including urine leaks, pelvic pain, and prolapse. Pelvic floor muscles have been proven to benefit from yoga, an ancient discipline that combines physical postures, breathing techniques, and meditation to aid in the relaxation and stretching of muscles.

The positive effects of yoga include:

- **Strengthening the pelvic floor muscles**

Yoga practices that involve engaging the core and pelvic floor muscles, such as the boat pose (Navasana), the bridge pose (Setu Bandhasana), and the chair pose (Utkatasana) involve contracting and engaging the pelvic floor muscles. These poses could be held for a few breaths, building strength over time and can help strengthen the pelvic floor muscles. Yoga can ease pelvic floor pain, strengthen and stabilize the pelvic floor muscles, and even help women regain control over their urination. Also, there's evidence showing that yoga can help lower prolapse risk and enhance sexual performance. By including breathwork, yoga can also help the pelvic floor become stronger. Exercises that engage and develop the pelvic floor muscles include the breath of fire and ujjayi breathing. We will practice these a bit later.

- **Improved awareness of the pelvic floor muscles**

One of the main advantages of yoga is that it can help you become more conscious of your pelvic muscles. Your instructor will encourage you to concentrate on breathing and become more aware of your bodily feelings. Awareness is the first step to improving the pelvic floor muscles' condition. You can increase your awareness of your pelvic floor muscles, including where they are located and what they do, by practicing mindfulness and breathwork. Some yoga poses, and exercises can also help people by increasing awareness, isolating, and engaging the pelvic floor muscles. For instance, the pigeon position (Kapotasana) calls for you to relax your pelvic floor muscles, while the bridge pose (Setu Bandhasana) calls for you to contract them. Anyone can benefit from the positions and exercises.

- **Improved blood flow**

Yoga positions that include twisting and inversions, like the triangle posture (Trikonasana) and the shoulder stand (Sarvangasana), or Legs up the Wall help improve blood flow to the pelvic area. By reversing the forces of gravity on the body, these positions help the pelvic organs and muscles receive more blood and nutrients. Moreover, yoga breathing techniques like "ocean breath" or ujjayi breathing might enhance blood flow to the pelvic floor muscles. Ujjayi breathing can encourage blood flow and nutrients to the pelvic area by boosting oxygenation and circulation.

There are many advantages of increased blood flow to the pelvic floor muscles including:

- Enhancing the health and performance of the pelvic muscles and organs.

- Minimizing pain and discomfort.

- Enhancing general well-being.

To practice Ujjayi breathing:

You inhale through your nose and exhale through your nose. The emphasis is in your throat. You constrict the back of your throat slightly, as if you are breathing through a straw, which creates an ocean sound or a soft snoring sound. Be mindful of relaxing your jaw, neck and throat. We unconsciously hold a lot of tension here. Keep in mind this breath can produce heat in your body. There may be times when you want a more restorative and relaxing practice or if you are pregnant, you may just choose to hold the intention of the breath rather than physically practice.

Improved flexibility of the pelvic floor muscles

Yoga poses, for example, the pigeon pose (*Kapotasana*) and the happy baby pose (*Ananda Balasana*), can increase flexibility by loosening and releasing pelvic floor muscles. The pigeon pose involves relaxing the pelvic floor muscles while extending the hip flexors and glutes. As a result, the pelvic floor muscles can relax and increase their range of motion. The happy baby pose involves grabbing the feet and pushing the knees toward the chest while you are on your back. In addition to stretching the pelvic floor muscles, this pose stretches the hips, inner thighs, and groin. Reduced pelvic pain and discomfort, better posture, and increased mobility can result from increased flexibility in the pelvic floor area.

Consistent yoga practice can help prevent related health issues in the pelvic muscles and help maintain pelvic floor health.

Improvement of posture

Yoga helps with posture, which could positively affect the pelvic floor muscles. The pelvic floor muscles may become tense due to poor posture, which can worsen pelvic irritation and functionality. When people have good posture, the pelvis' weight is distributed evenly, and the pelvic floor muscles are in their normal position. By doing so, the pelvic floor muscles may experience less strain and perform more effectively.

Rehabilitation after birth

Pelvic floor muscles are under continuous stress and trauma throughout the entire period of pregnancy and childbirth. After pregnancy, it is recommendable to practice yoga to help rehabilitate the pelvis and resume normal body functions.

In conclusion, the pelvic floor is very important in women's overall well-being. Practicing yoga regularly could help maintain, heal, and rehabilitate a strained pelvic floor for better health. The health of the pelvic floor muscles can benefit from yoga's emphasis on physical postures, breathing techniques, and meditation. Adding yoga into one's daily routine can be a very helpful tool to preserve the pelvic floor muscles' health and functionality and promote general physical well-being. Additionally, for your mental well-being, breathing, and meditation helps in clearing your thoughts and building a positive mentality. Yoga does not only have a positive effect on bodily function but also on psychological function.

Hatha yoga in urology: Hypertonicity and hypo-tonicity of muscles

It has been discovered that practicing Hatha yoga, a style of yoga that emphasizes physical postures, breathing exercises, and meditation, is useful for urological problems. The back and pelvis's musculoskeletal, neurological, and myofascial function is linked to chronic urological illnesses like interstitial cystitis, vulvodynia, prostatodynia, arthralgia, and incontinence. To treat symptoms like urinary incontinence, pelvic discomfort, and sexual dysfunction, yoga can help strengthen and relax the pelvic floor muscles, essential to urological health.

There are two main forms of pelvic floor dysfunction: pelvic floor hypertonicity and hypotonicity.

Pelvic floor hypotonicity

Muscle weakness or a lack of tone is referred to as hypotonicity. This describes the pelvic floor in terms of the muscles' inability to effectively carry out their duties, such as supporting the pelvic organs. Urinary incontinence, pelvic organ prolapse, and trouble executing some yoga poses that call for strong pelvic floor muscles are all symptoms of pelvic floor hypotonicity. It can be treated using asanas that strengthen the superficial layer of the urethral and anal sphincters and the deep layer, or levator ani, of the pelvic floor muscles. Yoga postures like the bridge, cobra, and chair pose that emphasize strengthening the pelvic floor muscles may benefit those with hypotonicity. The pelvic floor muscles' capacity to support the pelvic organs and manage fecal and urine continence can be improved with the help of these poses. Yoga positions can also help tonify the muscles in the pelvic floor by focusing on good alignment and using the core muscles.

Pelvic floor hypertonicity

This condition has an excessive increase in muscle tone, and it can lead to muscle stiffness, pain, and reduced range of motion. Pelvic muscles can become hypertonic due to various factors, for example, chronic stress, childbirth, or poor posture. The hypertonicity of the pelvic floor muscles can be reduced with specific asanas and breathing techniques. For instance, the pelvic floor muscles can be relaxed and tension reduced by using deep breathing techniques like diaphragmatic breathing. Similarly, performing asanas like bound angle posture and garland pose can help stretch and relieve tension in the pelvic floor muscles.

Yet, additional hatha yoga poses and breathing exercises might make the pelvic floor muscles more hypertonic. For example, if performed wrongly, root lock and the abdominal lock might result in an increase in pelvic floor muscle tension. Similar to how the extended holding of some poses can result in hypertonicity of the pelvic floor muscles.

In conclusion, Hatha yoga can be an effective treatment for urological issues brought on by hyper- and hypotonicity of the pelvic floor. Yoga can assist in increasing muscle tone, reducing stress, and improving the pelvic floor's ability to support the pelvic organs and regulate continence by focusing on specific muscle groups and using breathing methods. However, it is crucial to practice yoga under a certified instructor's supervision to ensure that the proper poses and techniques are followed to prevent further injury or a worsening of pre-existing conditions. Consequently, practicing yoga can significantly enhance medical treatment by enhancing myofascial function and musculoskeletal alignment.

Yoga poses (*asanas*) to help strengthen pelvic floor muscles

Yoga postures can effectively strengthen the pelvic floor muscles, which are essential for urological health. Any rotation or dysfunction in the lower back or bony pelvis will also lead to sickness because the pelvic floor and these structures operate together. As a result, the asanas for pelvic yoga also contain postures that can be used to strengthen, stretch, and maintain the primary muscles that affect the pelvic structure in balance.

Here are poses that are important in strengthening the pelvis:

- Frog pose (*Malasana pose*)

- Bridge pose (*Setu Bandhasana*)

- Plank pose

- Bird pose

- Chair pose (Utkatasana)

- The warrior pose (Virabhadrasana)

- Mountain pose (*Tadasana*)

- Reclining twist (*Supta Matsyendrasana*)

- Reclining bound angle pose (*Supta Baddha Konasana*)

- Child's pose (*balasana*)

- Cobra pose

- Cow pose

- Cat pose

- Crocodile pose

Customized yoga programs

Yoga is like any other physical exercise used for therapy and must always be planned and worked in relation to the individual's medical history. The first stage in creating a yoga program specifically for pelvic dysfunctions is to evaluate the individual's condition and requirements. A consultation with a medical specialist and a session with a certified yoga therapist who focuses on pelvic health can accomplish this. Before beginning, the doctor and the yoga instructor should assess the patient's body type and weight, age, general health, level of physical fitness, and any prior surgical conditions, such as difficult births, bladder suspensions, hysterectomies, or any prostate operations.

The yoga program can be customized to the individual's condition based on the evaluation, considering any limitations or contraindications. It is best to design a therapeutic yoga program for a person with a chronic illness that addresses their physical and emotional needs rather than blindly beginning one. For instance, certain poses that put pressure on the pelvic area may need to be avoided if the person has pelvic pain. Exercises that concentrate on relaxing and strengthening the pelvic floor muscles may be added if the person has pelvic floor muscle dysfunction.

Once a person's fundamental physical condition has been taken care of, a yoga program can be designed to allow them to minimize their symptoms in the comfort of their own homes. Yoga doesn't require specialized equipment, heavy lifting, or a lot of money.

The fundamentals of every effective program are followed by a good basic yoga program: warm-up exercises, primary exercises, and cool-down activities. Deep breathing exercises are one way that yoga differs from other forms of exercise. Breathing exercises are crucial because they promote oxygenation, which encourages the release of endorphins while also assisting in stress reduction and cardiovascular function.

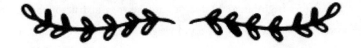

Effects of pregnancy and childbirth on pelvic floor muscles

The complicated female pelvic floor support system comprises the pelvic floor muscles and connective tissue. The levator ani muscle, one of the primary supporting muscles, and the coccyx muscle are the two main pelvic floor muscles among them. Fascia and ligaments make up the pelvic floor's connective tissue, and the pelvic floor muscles work with the connective tissue to form a "hanging net" that supports the pelvic organs in their proper place.

The pelvic floor muscles can be significantly impacted by childbirth. Sadly, some parts of childbirth have not been studied for their potential impact. Moreover, extensive and proper research on the effects of childbirth on pelvic muscle function after the first few weeks following delivery is yet to be done.

Pregnant women's bodies undergo some changes, including the uterus' expansion and the release of relaxin hormone which affects the pelvic floor muscles. The weight of the uterus steadily increases as the growing fetus in the womb does. As a result, the neutral axis shifts forward and the waist and abdomen protrude forward, putting pressure on the pelvic floor. Although the pelvic floor muscle has a certain degree of elasticity due to the prolonged nature of pregnancy and the constant and intense pressure placed on it, prolonged pressure and load will damage the elasticity of the pelvic floor muscle and impair its toughness. Pelvic floor muscle fibers get deformed as a result, which reduces muscle strength. The pelvic floor muscles weaken and stretch out, which can cause some pelvic floor dysfunctions, including pelvic organ prolapse, fecal incontinence, and urine incontinence.

The pelvic floor muscles may also be impacted by the delivery method. When a woman has a vaginal delivery, the pelvic floor muscles may get further stretched or torn as the baby passes the birth canal. This is particularly true when the birth is challenging or if the baby is big. Injuries to the pelvic floor muscles after vaginal deliveries that use forceps or vacuum assistance also have a higher risk. Vaginal birth is linked to lower pelvic muscle strength than cesarean birth, according to several small studies on postpartum women. Nevertheless, even women with cesarean sections may experience pelvic floor muscle damage during pregnancy or labor.

Depending on the baby's size, the length of labor, the use of forceps or vacuum, the woman's age, and general health, the degree of pelvic floor muscle damage can differ from woman to woman. While some women may experience mild to moderate pelvic floor muscle damage that eventually goes away on its own, other women may need therapy, including pelvic floor exercises, to rebuild their muscles' strength and functionality.

Neurogenic and pelvic floor dysfunction may result from myogenic damage. Both acute and long-term alterations may harm the pelvic floor muscles. Age and various childbirth-related conditions will gradually worsen the irreversible alterations brought on by pelvic floor damage, leading to pelvic floor dysfunction. After giving birth, women who experience pelvic floor dysfunctions should get therapy from a medical expert, such as a pelvic floor physical therapist, who may create a treatment plan specifically for them. Rehabilitative yoga can also be considered, but a yoga expert should be consulted.

The physiological effects of yoga

The mental health of postpartum women has recently been the subject of domestic and foreign studies. According to a study done in Hungary, pregnant women had a risk of postpartum depression of about 12–16%. Depression in pregnant women is correlated with their serum hydrocortisone levels. Low birth weight risk is increased by a persistently elevated hydrocortisone level in the serum. The American Academy of Obstetrics and Gynecology advises healthcare providers to monitor the mental health of their postpartum patients. Non-pharmacological therapies should be started immediately for people with psychological problems.

Yoga can be used in place of or in addition to other exercises to strengthen the pelvic floor muscles. It may reduce depression, stress, and anxiety while helping people manage their medical conditions, which can boost mental health and overall quality of life. Yoga, one of the world's oldest practices for maintaining health, has special appeal and characteristics. It prioritizes the oneness and harmony between the body and mind, in contrast to other fitness regimens that place greater emphasis on physical activities. Asanas, awareness, and breathing are all combined in yoga, which helps to exercise and relax a person's physical and psychological elements. Yoga practitioners can determine the right intensity and load based on a given set of circumstances. The motions and postures are calm and gentle. Yoga is suitable for postpartum mothers with various physical issues because of this. Meditation is an integral part of yoga practice and helps individuals focus on positive things, reduce distracting thoughts, relieve stress, alleviate fatigue and symptoms of depression.

Postpartum depression is thought to be improved by yoga via several physiological pathways, The hypothalamic-pituitary-adrenal (HPA) axis is prone to an imbalance in postpartum women with depression, and elevated cortisol levels are another factor. According to a randomized controlled trial, yoga can lessen the HPA axis's stress response and lower blood cortisol levels, which may help with the symptoms of depression. Second, research has shown that yoga helps control neurotransmitters like norepinephrine, serotonin, and dopamine, which are linked to depression, even though the mechanism is poorly understood. Yoga has been shown to raise dopamine and GABA levels in the brain, indicating that it may be a useful treatment for depression.

Last, depression frequently results in sleep disruptions such as increased REM sleep intensity and shallow sleep depth. Yoga has been shown to enhance sleep quality, especially for people with chronic insomnia and the elderly. As a result, it is hypothesized that yoga may lessen depression symptoms in postpartum women by enhancing their sleep.

Ultimately, postpartum depression is a significant global issue in women's mental health. Thankfully, non-pharmacological treatments, like yoga, present a viable substitute for postpartum mothers experiencing psychological issues. Yoga can improve the overall quality of life by reducing stress, anxiety, and sadness symptoms. With its emphasis on the harmony and unification of the body and mind, yoga can be a great workout program for postpartum women suffering from various physical challenges. It can help postpartum women who are depressed by regulating many physiological processes, such as the HPA axis and neurotransmitters. Yoga can also help improve sleep quality, which is typically disturbed by depression.

Chapter Six

Womb Awareness and Healing

S urprisingly, we are all products of the womb, the least known part of our body. Many of us don't think too much about it until something happens or doesn't happen, for example, waiting for the monthly period to arrive. It is a place with immense power, but it's ignored, neglected, and forgotten by many of us. The womb is not just a place to give birth to babies. It's a place that births us, with new realities and holds power for deep transformation. It is a place of death, life, and possibilities, and its power has been appreciated for thousands of years. A womb is a place where our bodies store different types of traumas, whether physical, emotional, or energetic.

As women, many of us believe that the womb is also the source of our womanhood, including our sensuality, sexuality, self-esteem, and other aspects of femininity. The womb space is our source of inner strength and creativity. It is where we give the planet new life or new ideas. The fact is that giving birth doesn't always manifest as a child in the physical realm. On an energetic level, every one of us goes through the process of giving birth to a new idea, venture, purpose, or even way of life. We may feel stuck if energetic blocks develop in this area (our sacral chakra). Without a free flow of Shakti (feminine energy), we lack clarity and have limited strength. Our wombs are direct entry points for spirit into the physical world, whether it takes the shape of a child or the inspiration to bring an idea to life.

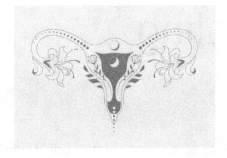

The wounding womb

A developing fetus is entirely reliant on the mother it resides inside of. A mother who abuses drugs or alcohol causes significant harm to her offspring because the fetus is connected to the mother using the umbilical cord and gets air, food, water, and whatever else the mother digests. A fetus gets from its mother more than just nutrition and chemical input. A mother's emotional state, internal environment, and exterior environment are all very perceptible to the fetus as well as to the mother herself.

Fetuses also experience adverse consequences while inside the mother's body for nine months. They absorb toxins like nicotine, bio-chemicals like adrenaline, and over-the-counter or prescribed medications, some of which can cause congenital disabilities, loud noises, toxic fumes, food with low nutritional value, violent behavior, and strong emotions of rage and anger because they share a bloodstream with their mothers. Since so many substances can pass through the placenta, it is no longer regarded as a reliable barrier that protects a baby.

It's important to remember that not all ancestral trauma dates back several centuries. Some of it was passed down through your experiences while in the wombs of your mother and even your grandmother. Whether you actively recall it or not, this formative period molded you in many ways, changing your DNA, emotional state, and psychological well-being. Following traumatic experiences like assault and rape, it was discovered that the children of such mothers "had a significantly higher rate of developing serious psychological problems." (Source: Rachel Yehuda, Ph.D., Professor of Psychiatry and Neuroscience). This is proof from science that family trauma is passed down through generations. It also demonstrates stress's strong impact on us while we are still in our mother's womb.

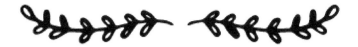

Techniques for Womb Healing

We had no control over our experience as fetuses. Still, as individuals who are opting to let go of the unfavorable narrative our bodies hold, we can now write a new script.

Here's how we can do that:

Through Imagination

This helps you imagine yourself in a different state, such as imagining yourself as a **Loving Woman**. Through imagination, you get to imagine a scene that implies you are whole and loving now. When you come from a state of love, it bypasses a lot of the negative thought patterns and behaviours that keep us stuck in the past, blaming, and being the "victim." When you know that you are love and you let that lead you in your interactions, disposition, and relationships, the transformation is your life is amazing. This starts in the imagination, trying on a new state of Loving Woman, and letting her lead the way. You can embody this position where it could be possible to remember and change how things turn out. You basically revise the past story and make it better. You can approach this playfully and see your situation from a different perspective, and this can be life-changing to many, especially those suffering from traumatic experiences. Take a short trip to your mind and then to the womb as a fetus through imagining to create a healthier and happier time in the womb, bringing the images shaped by your fetal brain into conscious awareness.

Art therapy

It uses the creative process of art-making to improve and enhance the emotional and mental health of individuals of all ages. It is associated with the belief that the creative process involved in artistic assertiveness helps people resolve conflicts and problems, manage behavior, develop self-awareness, achieve insight, and develop self-control over emotions. The mental images can offer solutions to problems and insights into the cause of the problem. Most sessions focus on your inner experience –feeling, perception, and imagination. Art therapy helps you visualize what's going on in the mind and learn new ways to change thinking patterns which can lead to a new perspective.

Dance movement therapy

Dance therapy makes use of movement to enhance both emotional and physical health. It has recently been rediscovered as a method of overcoming stress by enabling people to communicate without using words. We already know that trauma impacts both the body and the brain in different ways.

Dance/Movement Therapy (D/MT) provides changes in the sensorimotor experience that support self-regulation, memory processing, and success in daily life for persons who have traumatic experiences. The body retains the memory of a traumatic incident by repeating thoughts and patterns that continuously replay the horrific incident as if it were on a loop, affecting neurological processing. Those who experience these effects typically get "top-down" therapeutic methods that prioritize verbal communication before understanding physical input. It is frequently impossible and unwise for someone with memory loss to try to remember the event. Art, music, drama, and dance act as a translator to the speechlessness that comes with terror and fragmented memories.

Dance/movement therapy aims to establish safety and reconnect you with your body to identify patterns and conditioned responses. D/MT can be used as a "bottom-up" therapeutic processing, Utilizing the connection between the mind and body to work together as one helps in the exchange and flow of information, processing it in a bidirectional circuit to regulate the internal systems of the individual.

Focusing on the body of the client and therapist in D/MT can produce a change in the client's unconscious body reaction, as well as a reaction in conscious psychological processes. If the body constantly replays what the mind has repressed, then new movement patterns can help the mind re-focus and calm the aroused response systems. Increasing the range of movement patterns within the body is a way of introducing new behaviors. Per movement theorists, movement increases the range of action and interaction.

Somatic therapy

Somatic therapy is derived from the Greek word soma, which means body. The concept of "somatic healing therapies" refers particularly to those treatments that take a bottom-up approach and are included in the category of mind-body therapies. This psychotherapy method uses the body's awareness as a potent tool and intervention during therapies. Somatic methods are used to explore the relationship between the mind, body, brain, and behavior. Therapists use somatic training interventions to facilitate their patients' healing by calming the nervous system. Examples of somatic therapy could include breathing, self touch practices, and grounding techniques.

Sensual Somatic TM Embodiment

This practice is close to my heart. I completed a 3-month immersion and certification to facilitate this beautiful practice and it was life changing. Sensual Somatic TM is a practice of sensual dance and somatic healing. It is a practice to drop into the body, develop awareness of sensations and feelings, and find your own language of body movement through dance and yoga. Much of the practice includes self touch to regulate the nervous system. On a deep level, embracing, exploring, and expression of our own unique sensuality allows us to bring deep seated sexual traumas to the surface and heal them. Personally, I developed a greater sense of internal and external boundaries as I developed greater somatic awareness and trust. This has been revolutionary for me in my relationship to myself and others, as well as my sexual healing. Go to resources section for additional support.

The concept of the earth being feminine

A large part of any somatic or yoga practice is connecting, grounding, and releasing to the earth. Have you ever wondered why we call her Mother Earth?

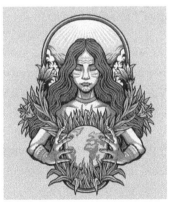

Depiction of Mother Earth

In ancient Mesoamerican culture, the idea of the earth as feminine reflected the significance of the natural world in supporting life and the notion that the earth played a strong and protective role in people's lives. Sweat baths and caves served as entrances to this feminine realm, metaphorically compared to the vagina and womb of the earth mother. As a result, they were closely linked to the complexities of female fecundity and earth deities such as childbirth.

The idea that the earth is feminine is widespread throughout Mesoamerica and is specifically present in the belief system of North America. The earth's entrances serve as metaphors for the female form, and water that emerges from the earth is conceptually linked to a woman's genital fluids. Similar to how female vaginal fluids appear, caves are frequently thought of as sources of terrestrial waters. Sweat baths were commonly referred to as "flower houses." They were employed in healing practices by midwives and healers connected to the goddesses and often used aromatic herbs to treat various illnesses and facilitate childbirth. And because reproduction and childbirth are messy, bathing the infant was crucial to sanitize them and eliminate the parent's filth from their sexual activities.

The Aztec, Maya, and Olmec cultures, which are all part of Mesoamerica, all had unique views on and reverence for the earth as a feminine force. The goddess Coatlicue served as the personification of the Earth in Aztec mythology.

She was frequently portrayed as a terrifying figure wearing a pendant made of human hearts and a skirt made of serpents.

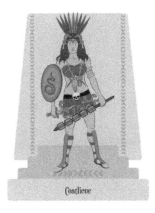

Coatlicue

As the mother of all gods and people, this image represented her control over life and mortality. The earth was said to have been made by Coatlicue from her own body, and she was regarded as a symbol of the duality of life, death, and creation and destruction.

Tlaltecuhtli, a goddess connected to the earth and fertility in Aztec mythology, was another significant figure. She was frequently portrayed as a terrifying woman with a serpent's head. Her breasts represented mountains, her hair grass and vegetation, and her torso was pictured as the earth's crust. Tlaltecuhtli was viewed as a strong and nurturing force in charge of sustaining life on earth and fostering the development of crops. The deity Ixchel served as the personification of the Earth in Maya mythology. She was frequently portrayed as a young lady with a skirt and a feathered headdress because she was connected to fertility, water, and the moon. Ixchel was revered as a goddess of childbirth and weaving who could bring rain and fertility to the country. She was also associated with weaving. The Maya thought it was their responsibility to take care of and protect the earth because they saw it as a living being.

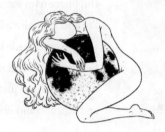

A deep reverence for the earth as a feminine power was also shared by the Olmec civilization, which predates the Aztecs and Mayans. The "Great Mother," a deity worshipped by the Olmecs, was connected to the natural cycles and the development of crops. The "Great Mother" was frequently portrayed as a pregnant woman to represent her position as the originator of life.

Ancient Mesoamerican cultures recognized the natural world's value in sustaining life, mirrored in their conception of the earth as feminine. These societies had extensive agriculture and depended on the soil to survive. They thought it was their responsibility to respect and preserve the natural world because they understood the earth's capacity to provide food, water, and other resources. The Mesoamerican civilizations viewed the earth as a potent and nurturing force capable of producing and supporting life. The feminine side of the earth was viewed as a source of sustenance and nourishment because it was connected to fertility, development, and the natural cycles. The Mesoamerican cultures also progressed in understanding agriculture, environmental practices, and spiritual beliefs. They created intricate irrigation systems, terraced fields, and crop rotation practices, all of which made it possible for them to grow crops effectively and sustainably. Additionally, they had a thorough knowledge of nature's cycles, which allowed them to forecast weather patterns and organize their agricultural practices accordingly.

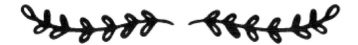

Practical Exercises for Womb Healing and Pelvic Floor Strengthening

How to do a Kegel

A Kegel is very much the same as root lock or *Mul bandh* in yoga.

First, exhale, and then contract the anus, as if you are holding in a bowel movement. Then, add in the contraction of the sexual organ which can feel like stopping the flow of urine. The contraction of the perineal muscles is a kegel. Finally when we are practicing root lock, you additionally pull in the navel point by drawing in the lower abdomen to the spine. Inhale and release the contraction. *Mul* means "root, base, or source." *Bandh* means "lock." For women: During the heavy part of menses, and after the third month of pregnancy, do not do strenuous yoga or root lock. Later I will specify which yoga poses to avoid.

The Kegel myths

In this era of information, we are constantly bombarded with advice on how best to live our lives and what to do with our bodies. But no information can run its course without having some rumors, and Kegels are no exception. Even as an adult, you might still hold to some Kegel myths you didn't know have no supporting evidence.

Due to the Kegel exercise's growing popularity, it is simple to believe that any problem involving the pelvic floor muscles can be "fixed" by performing these exercises. This supposition is further supported by many businesses that enthusiastically promote fancy Kegel products and devices to people seeking symptom relief. In reality, pelvic floor pain is frequently more complicated than many realize.

Below are some of the myths associated with Kegels;

1. Kegels are the best way to strengthen the pelvic floor: While Kegels can be an effective way to strengthen the pelvic floor muscles, they are not the only or the best way. Other functional exercises, such as squats, lunges, and bridges, provide better activation of these muscles compared to conventional Kegels. Additionally, it's important to address any underlying issues contributing to pelvic floor weakness, such as obesity or chronic coughing.

2. Practice Kegels by stopping urine: While it's true that stopping the flow of urine can be useful in identifying muscles involved in a Kegel, it's not advisable to do Kegels while urinating. This leads to urine backflow into the urethra leading to increased risks of urinary tract infections. It probably won't hurt to stop urine to identify pelvic floor muscle, but making a habit out of it just might. It's best to practice Kegels

in a comfortable position, such as lying down and without any distractions.

3. It would be best to do at least 100 Kegels daily: it is important to note that not everyone needs to do Kegels, and the number of Kegels you need to do varies from person to person. Starting out slowly is crucial, and as your muscles get stronger, you should progressively increase the number of repetitions. Too many Kegels performed too quickly can result in muscle fatigue and may not have long-term effects.

4. Do Kegels everywhere: Kegels can be performed discreetly, but doing them in a relaxed posture is crucial. While standing or moving around performing Kegels, you might be unable to engage your pelvic floor muscles due to distractions. It's best to perform Kegels in a calm, private setting like your home or a private room.

Kegel weights

Kegel weights are tiny weights that are inserted into the vagina. They are also commonly known as vagina balls. Although they have been used for many years, they have recently become trendy and fashionable. Many people in ancient China thought that having strong pelvic floor muscles and vaginal muscles would increase their life force energy. Archaeologists have found Jade eggs shaped like ancient Kegel weights, and even intricate renaissance drawings show how they were used in the past. Jade eggs, also known as yoni eggs, are weights in the form of eggs made of the natural crystal that was widely used in ancient China. They are still used today.

They can help you recover from childbirth, reduce pelvic prolapse, help with urine incontinence, and even improve hip and back pain for some people. They also play a role in improving your sex life since a strong pelvic muscle increases sexual pleasure, and they are also used as sex toys by some couples.

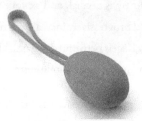

Kegel weight

Kegel weights are made to fit like a weighted tampon and easily slide into the vaginal canal. Once inside, the pelvic floor muscles contract to hold the Kegel weight in position while wrapping around it, providing resistance training. While some women prefer to hold the weights in place for 10–20 minutes each day while they rest or perform simple domestic tasks, others enjoy practicing the contraction and relaxation phases of Kegel exercises while using Kegel weights.

Kegel weight proponents claim that all of them can strengthen and retrain your pelvic floor muscles, but they vary in effectiveness, size, weight, technology, the substance used to make them, and value for money.

Kegel balls vary in size and weight; they weigh between 10 and 100 grams. Just like any other strength training weight, starting light and increasing the weight gradually as your muscles develop is advisable. Insert the Kegel weights into your vagina like a tampon after washing and lubricating them (use water-based lubricant if you feel lubricant is necessary). Try standing up as a possible posture. Holding onto the attached rope, place the weight into the slot. After it's been put in, contract your pelvic floor muscles. Relax and do not forget to breathe. You will sense it lifting away from your hand when it is on the string. Try to hold this weight while standing still with your muscles tensed for a few minutes. If this is too challenging, you can work while sitting. You can advance to the next weight when you can maintain the current weight for at least 15 minutes over two to three days. Ensure that you can hold the current weight for some time before moving on to the next weight.

Keep them clean after every session.

The best Kegel weights are made from body-safe silicon, are easy to clean, and should come with varying resistance levels for when the pelvic floor muscles develop or become stronger. Avoid cheap ones since most of them could be made of harmful plastics that expose vaginal tissues to toxins and chemical coloring that can irritate them.

Below are some examples of Kegel balls;

- Secret Whispers Kegel training kit

- INTIMINA intimina laselle

- LELO Beads

- We-Vibe Bloom

- Je Joue 3-step Progressive Kegel Kit

- Intimate Rose Kegel Exercise Weights

Please do enough research before purchasing the above or any other type of Kegel balls.

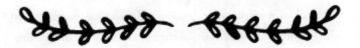

Tools for healing your womb

Did you know that your womb can be restored to its pure, unadulterated form? Using intuitive healing methods in conjunction with energy work, bodywork, diet, herbal remedies, and lifestyle medicine, you can effectively release emotional blocks, womb-born trauma, and historical imprints left by prior lovers. Womb healing can support mental recovery from losses like miscarriage, stillbirth, and abortions and assist in cutting energy cords of attachment.

Below are some of the tools I have used in healing my womb.

Yoni eggs

Kegel balls, yoni eggs, jade eggs...Despite their many varied names, most of them share a common nature. Yoni eggs are simply crystals carved into an egg's shape. They have been in use for thousands of years in many parts of Asia. They are used to promote sensuality and strengthen and heal the vaginal muscle, and they are placed inside the vaginal canal. The stone tones the pelvic floor muscles, which also helps in bladder control, lubrication, libido, and postpartum healing.

Yoni is a Sanskrit word with many meanings, the most common one being the vagina or vaginal area. They are made of various crystals, commonly clear quartz, jade, and rose quartz, each type of crystal serving a specific purpose. The use of crystals allows the metaphysical healing properties to bring healing and nurturing, cleansing, and cleaning to the yoni and womb space.

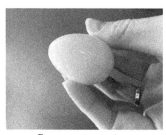

Rose quartz yoni egg

Yoni eggs come in two basic types, drilled and non-drilled. The drilled yoni is attached to a string for easy removal from the vagina. They are the most popular since they address the widespread fear of being impossible to retrieve or getting stuck in the vagina. Some women retain the eggs for 3+ weeks with no issues. Drilled eggs can be hard to clean since they have holes. The non-drilled ones are ideal. If you plan to attach weight to your eggs, ensure you are vigilant in your hygiene to avoid bacteria or yeast infections. The contraindication for yoni egg use is if you have an intrauterine device (IUD).

They also come in different sizes, and it's advisable to start from the large to the small one. That's because the small size can be more challenging because they need stronger vaginal muscles to hold them in place.

Types of Yoni eggs

Below is a list of some of these crystals used to create yoni eggs

- **Jade eggs**

The most popular yoni egg type is unquestionably the jade egg; some people mistakenly refer to the complete assortment as various types of jade eggs! These stones are said to give off a bright, healing energy that aids in cleansing the body, speeds up wound recovery, and harmonizes the user's mood. Additionally, it is a potent charm that draws tranquility, longevity, inventiveness, and wisdom. Jade eggs can assist in removing negativity and increasing calming feelings. They also help support the heart chakra while helping in pursuing inner desires and igniting passion.

Jade eggs are frequently recommended to people who are more concerned with developing and improving their pelvic floor muscles because of these qualities. Jade is believed to have been used for thousands of years.

- **Black obsidian**

This crystal, purported to be the stone of truth, is the most frequently used in crystal balls. It aids in the illumination of secrets and the attainment of decision-making clarity. Obsidian is also powerful enough to tap into your negative emotions and slowly absorb the negative energies, another characteristic that is frequently attributed to it. This makes obsidian yoni eggs a great option for those trying to overcome a traumatic experience or deal with challenging negative emotions.

It connects to the root chakra. Obsidian is a dependable stone and an effective ally for releasing emotions and trauma trapped in the body, particularly in the pelvis. It transforms negative energy and aids in treating some bodily conditions that affect women's bodies.

- **Rose quartz**

It is a crystal that derives its name from its lovely rose-pink color. This crystal is available in a variety of stunning rose hues. It radiates a potent vibration of unwavering love, pleasure, warmth, and healing, which is why it's also called the "love stone." It is commonly linked with love and romance issues and is called the "heart-healing crystal." The heart chakra and the thymus chakra, which are linked to compassion, both resonate with the strong energy of this lovely pink rose quartz crystal yoni egg. Additionally, it aids in overcoming all forms of trauma and anxiety. People frequently use rose quartz to aid their emotional and tough breakup recovery. Alternatively, other people use it when they are trying to get into a partnership right now or open themselves up to more love.

Yoni eggs and the pelvic floor

Yoni eggs help a woman develop a respectful, kind, and therapeutic connection with her pelvic floor. Our intimate relationship with our partner is impacted by the quality of our sex life, which is influenced by our pelvic health. We must take a closer look at what's happening because when this aspect of our lives is compromised, the general quality of life suffers.

Here are ways yoni eggs impact the pelvic floor;

Yoni egg enthusiasts assert that they have both bodily and spiritual advantages. Physically, it is believed that entering a yoni egg causes your body to perform an unintentional Kegel, thereby bolstering the pelvic floor.

Although using a yoni egg requires you to tighten your vaginal muscles, which can hurt you continuously, pelvic floor exercises have been shown to strengthen the muscles in the pelvic floor. Long-term pelvic floor contractions can cause those muscles to become more tense and difficult to release.

Yoni eggs help in increasing blood flow to the pelvic floor. The Yoni egg helps keep these muscles flexible, dexterous, and with life-force energy. Yoni eggs relax, soften the pelvic floor muscles, and tighten and tone the vagina.

Tantra and Kundalini

Historical context offers the most compelling explanation for the apparent contradiction in Indian attitudes toward sex. From writing the first works that treated sexual activity as a science to, more recently, being the source of the philosophical underpinnings of new-age groups' attitudes toward sex, India has played a major role in the history of sex. One could say that India was a pioneer in the use of sexual education through literature and art. As in all societies, there were differences in sexual behaviors between powerful rulers and the general populace in India. The latter frequently indulged in lifestyles that did not reflect accepted moral values. The demographic and socioeconomic conditions of India's multiethnic and multilingual communities vary greatly.

How did the idea that the feminine represents everything sexual come about? The phrase "*The female of the species is biologically and psy-*

chologically superior" was ingrained in the foundations of Aryan-Dravidian society and may have been an indirect acknowledgment of the phrase, which is now gnomic in Western sociology.

It is not only a notion in Eastern thought to personify as a female that manifests power and energy. The idea of feminine power is also deeply rooted within the racial consciousness of Western men. In the Hindu religion, women are viewed as the vessels of Shakti (power).

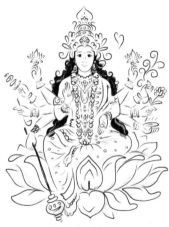

Goddess Shakti

This association with goddess Shakti recognizes women as the carriers of constructive and destructive forces. Hindu society struggles to reconcile the biological compulsion of these two potent forces, similar to many contemporary cultures.

Tantra is an ancient philosophical and spiritual tradition. The Tantra is derived from the Sanskrit word "tan" which means "enlargen," and "tra" which means "tools" or "instrument". Tantra, therefore, is a tool or instrument for expanding consciousness and achieving spiritual growth.

Tantra is often associated with the worship of the divine feminine. One of the key features of Tantra is its emphasis on the embodied experience. It sees the body as a vehicle for spiritual realization, recognizes the body as a source of pleasure and joy, and that these experiences can be used to deepen our connection to the divine.

Tantra is considered the most appropriate form of Kali Yuga, or Dark Age, because it explicitly acknowledges women as the greatest manifestation of God. One of the minor Upanishads quotes Tantra, says, *"the pubic hairs are the flames upon the altar, and the vulva is an altar."*

Tantra is the awakened Indian concept of how sex manifests physically. Tantra is still the most potent and important school of Indian thought, even though it is frequently misunderstood. Tantra is the origin of Indian metaphysics, even though Hinduism may be the mother of all ideologies. Swami Satyananda of Bihar, a modern-day Yogi, claims that Tantra, not Samkhya, is the intellectual foundation from which Yoga arose.

In Tantra, sexual energy is seen as a great force that can be harnessed for spiritual growth and transformation. The energy is known as Kundalini and is said to be lying coiled and dormant at the base of the spine and can be awakened and channeled through various practices.

Kundalini energy

Kundalini energy is the ideal life-force energy, an internal power source. It is also known as the serpent power in Hinduism. It is the source of our divine feminine vitality, spiritual abilities, and creative potential. You can practice Kundalini yoga to broaden awareness and achieve a state of lightness, joy, and limitless love. Kundalini causes an upward flow of energy and balances our chakras and energetic bodies by drawing the energy that is dormant at the base of our spines up to the top of our heads.

Using various postures, breathing, and sound techniques, the ultimate purpose of Kundalini Yoga is to free the Kundalini (serpent) power that is lying coiled and dormant at the base of our spine.

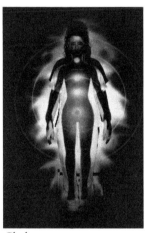

Kundalini Awakening involves drawing out the coiled Kundalini from its resting place and directing it upwards through the seven chakras or energy centers. When this dormant force of the Kundalini spreads freely upwards, you are taken to higher states of consciousness, and this process is called Kundalini Awakening.

Chakras or energy centers

For people practicing Kundalini techniques under the guidance of a competent, trained, and knowledgeable teacher, the experience includes feelings of bliss, unconditional love, and a sense of being connected with everything in the world. However, owing to misguidance and/or improper techniques, some people feel a sense of being under the influence of drugs, experience altered sleep patterns, and feel a sense of baseless fear. These spurious techniques have, unfortunately, made many Westerners wary of the "coiled serpent" and are fearful that if disturbed, it will strike them down.

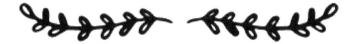

Orgasms

Orgasms are significant spiritually due to their ability to remove you from your head and into your body. You lose your ego, or the perception of being separate from the source, during an orgasm. Orgasm is also a very high-energy state, similar to an electrical current that runs from your genitalia through your spine and entire nervous system. The sexual chi energy from within gives you that "orgasmic glow" throughout the day.

Orgasms can bring you more than just pleasure in your bedroom. Regular orgasms play a very important role in our emotional and physical health and in achieving your desires.

Strong pelvic floor. Both males and women benefit from having a strong pelvic floor. By performing your Kegel movements regularly and engaging in regular sex, you can experience orgasms that last longer and are more intense. The advantages don't stop there, either. Women who have a strong pelvic floor have better bladder control and function.

Reducing pain. You might be relieved to discover that sex can actually lessen pain if you experience typical menstrual symptoms like cramps. An orgasm might be just what the doctor prescribed because endorphins and corticosteroids are released during an orgasm, which can help to reduce pain.

Regulates menstrual cycle. Did you realize that having sex frequently could help to control your menstrual cycle? Although many women struggle with irregular periods, few are aware that regular intercourse may be healthy. Women who have sex at least once per week have more regular cycles than those who have it infrequently or never, according to research from Stanford and Columbia colleges.

Practical Breathwork

Deep Belly Breathing or Womb Breathing

This is best done lying down, but you can also sit upright in a chair. Be sure your legs are uncrossed with feet flat on the floor. A really handy way I learned a visual aid with deep breathing in my yoga training was to hold a book against your belly as a visual for breath, but a hand on your belly or womb space works too.

Start by inhaling through your nose. Exhaling through your mouth.

Notice where your breath is in your body. Don't force it.

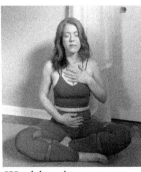

Womb breathing

Gradually you can start to lengthen and deepen the breath on the inhale and the exhale. As you inhale, you fill up your belly and will see your hand or the book push out gently. Imagine you are filling up your entire womb space with your breath. You continue to fill up your diaphragm, lungs, all the way up to your collarbone.

Then exhale the air out, down from your collarbone, lungs, and finally the belly drops back to its natural position as you empty the breath completely.

Repeat this for 10 breaths or more.

Alternate Nostril Breathing (Nadi Shodhana Pranayama)

Alternate nostril breathing reduces stress and shifts you from fight or flight mode into the parasympathetic nervous system where we feel relaxed and calm. *You may want to clear your nose with a tissue before beginning this practice.*

Sit comfortably with your spine as straight as possible.

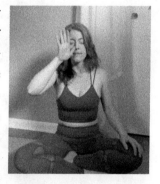

Rest your thumb on your right nostril and your index finger on your left nostril. Inhale deeply and exhale fully through your nose. Close the right nostril with your thumb and inhale through your left nostril. Close the left nostril with your index finger, open the right nostril (removing your thumb), and exhale through the right side.

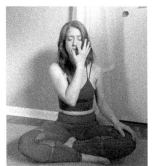

Pause briefly at the end of the exhale before inhaling through the right nostril. Close the right side with your thumb, open the left nostril (removing your index finger), and exhale through the left side. You have now completed one full cycle. Practice for 1-3 minutes.

Lion's Breath (Simha Pranayama)

1. Find a comfortable seated position in a space where you can feel comfortable making noise.

2. Inhale through your nose.

3. Open your mouth, stick out your tongue, extending it down toward your chin. It looks silly but this breath is really detoxifying and wonderful to regulate the emotions. Then forcefully exhale out your mouth, making a "ha" sound.

4. Relax your face between rounds and take a few normal breaths.

5. Practice for 5 rounds.

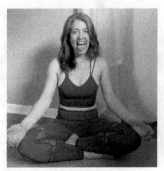

Lion's Breath

Breath of Fire

Breath of fire is a dynamic, energizing breath. You would not practice this breath when pregnant or menstruating or if you have had recent abdominal surgery or injury. Practice long deep breathing rather. With breath of fire, the emphasis is on the exhale.

You exhale powerfully through your nostrils and pull in the navel point. The inhale happens naturally when your belly relaxes back out. You go your own pace. With practice and experience, this breath can be fast, powerful and dynamic. You can start practicing up to 1 minute and work up from there.

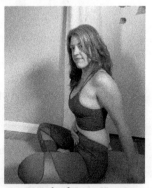

Breath of Fire - Keeping a hand on your belly can be helpful when learning and practicing this breath. Hand would come towards spine with the exhale.

Chapter Seven

Yoga for the Pelvic Floor

Stretches and Exercises for Daily Practice

H istorically, many have incorrectly defined yoga as a tool solely to benefit one's spiritual, religious, and psychological health. In recent decades, vigilant exploration has exposed the advantages of deep breathing (pranayama) and yoga positions (asanas), when practiced in modest exercise programs, on those affected by chronic disorders. Yoga is more than just physical exercise. Yoga means "union"; as such, it connects and unifies the mind, body, and spirit. This also means that when practicing the yoga asanas (the physical postures of yoga) we enjoy mental and physical benefits. With regular yoga practice comes more mindfulness, mental clarity, and self-awareness. It's common to feel more at peace and calm, even outside your yoga practice.

Yoga is an ancient practice, and it helps bring equilibrium to the mental, emotional, spiritual, and physical facets of your life, whether you are a beginner or a seasoned yogi. One of the greatest advantages of yoga is its ability to reduce pain while improving the overall quality of your life. Various yoga poses, like the cobra and warrior pose, can help reduce pelvic pain. Yoga can be a part of gynecological and pelvic pain treatment since it helps relieve and manage the pressure in your pelvic floor muscles.

There are no limits to the positive changes that you can gain. With a more restorative and restful type of yoga, you'll experience increased levels of relaxation from activating your body's resting state. A cardio-based yoga style promotes an increase in energy levels and vitality. Certain yoga poses improve balance and posture, whereas other poses help build muscle strength or improve flexibility and joint mobility. Many people tend to think of yoga as a last resort. However, this must be your first resort, especially before considering any pharmaceuticals. When properly diagnosing any ailment, having complete body awareness is quite important.

No doctor can tell you what your pain feels like, how the relief would feel, the tension you experience, or any other sensation you feel. You're the only one who can understand what you feel, and you're the only one who can gauge the sensations. When getting a proper diagnosis, it is essential to have all this inside. Yoga helps develop mindfulness and self-awareness. It encourages you and supports you in becoming more aware of what you feel and experience. You become the primary authority over your body by exploring, observing, and learning about yourself.

Regular practicing of yoga has both short- and long-term benefits. Although it may be difficult to incorporate yoga into your busy schedule, regular practice is necessary to see the positive change within yourself and achieve the desired results. But even practicing one longer sequence once a week or a shorter sequence every few days will improve your health and well-being.

But first, you'll need to identify and recognize your pelvic muscles. How can you do this?

Stop Test

The Stop Test is highly effective and should only be done until you can recognize your pelvic muscles. Stopping urination is unhealthy because it can snap bacteria into the urinary tract and interfere with the bladder-emptying mechanism. Do not try the Stop Test if you have a urinary tract or kidney infection. Never do the Stop Test more than once per day, either. Again, please ONLY do this if you have no awareness of your pelvic floor issues. Otherwise, the muscles you use to stop the flow of urine and hold in a bowel movement are your pelvic floor muscles. Do not get discouraged if you cannot stop urinating in the middle of the flow. With repeated effort, you will develop body awareness to isolate the correct muscles.

To perform this test:

- Sit on the toilet.

- Start urinating.

- Try to hold back urine for one to two seconds toward the end of the flow. Relax your body completely.

The muscles stopping the urine flow are the pelvic muscles. Learn to feel these muscles. Then finish urinating, completely emptying the bladder. The muscles you should focus on are the ones you feel tightening around your anus and urethra.

Practice squeezing these muscles when you are not urinating.

Finger test

- Sit on a chair or lie down.

- Put one or two fingers into the vagina.

- Squeeze and contract your muscles around the area as though you were holding back a bowel movement, lifting the vaginal walls into the pelvic cavity. You should be able to feel the muscles tighten around your fingers.

Medical exam

Another effective technique is to request a checkup from your doctor during your next gynecological exam to test you for pelvic strength and rate you on a scale of one through ten (one weakest, ten strongest). With the doctor's fingers inside you, contract your pelvic muscles and hold.

Once you've identified the muscles, try placing the flat of your palm over the midline of your pelvic region with your pubic bone centered under the palm and the fingers over the vaginal cavity. During the contraction of the muscles on the pelvic floor, you should feel a gentle "lift" of your pelvic muscles out of your hand. This will help you learn the feeling of isolating your pelvic floor muscles.

Yoga exercises for your pelvic floor

Here is where we will get into the yoga stretches that are especially good for strengthening the core and pelvic floor muscles, opening the hips and thighs, and also relaxing the pelvic floor muscles and feeling grounded.

Each pose has the accompanying Sanskrit name for your information. The poses are not in a specific order. With each pose I have specified if it is a grounding pose, core strengthening, hip opener, or standing pose. In the next chapter I give a few examples of sequences for these poses.

Mountain pose (*Tadasana*)

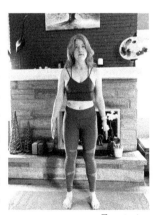

Mountain pose is a **grounding pose** and aligns the spine for better posture. While standing in mountain pose you can also contract your pelvic floor muscles. It seems simple but it's a very engaging pose. Stand with your feet parallel with knees facing straight ahead. Engage your leg muscles by pulling up from your feet and pelvis. Lengthen up the sides of your body and stand tall.

Front view

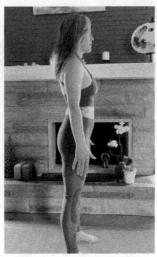

Side alignment of mountain pose

Feel lengthened and rooted into the earth. Take your shoulders back and bring your shoulder blades more onto your back. Breathe deeply here for several full breaths and then release.

Bird/dog pose *(Dandayamana Bharmanasana)* is excellent for strengthening the **core** muscles which surround the pelvic bowl.

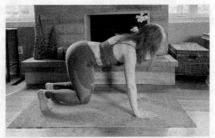

Dog pose, knees raised off the ground.

Start on your hands and knees with your hands directly underneath your shoulders and your knees underneath your hips for proper alignment. If possible, raise your knees slightly off the ground and float them a couple inches above the ground. Engage your core muscles.

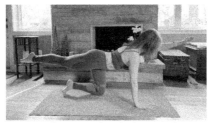

Left arm and right leg raised

This is called Dog pose. You can stay here for a minute and breathe deeply. You can lower your knees down for alternate leg and arm raises. Raise your right arm and left leg off the ground parallel to the ground.

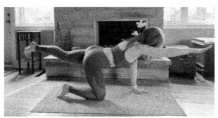

Alternate and raise right arm and left leg.

Then switch and raise the other alternate arm and leg. Inhale when you raise, exhale when you lower. Engage your core muscles and move slowly.

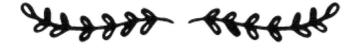

Bridge pose *(Setu Banda Sarvangasana)*

Start by lying on your back. Bridge pose is a **core** exercise. Bend your knees and bring your feet flat on the ground. Take a few deep breaths here.

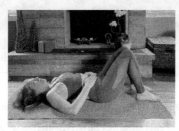

Prep pose. Taking a few deep breaths.

On the exhale, tilt your pelvis forward and articulate your lower spine on the floor. On the inhale, tilt your pelvis back. Continue the pelvic tilts. On the next exhale, articulate the spine to the ground and lift your hips into the air toward the sky. Hold here breathing deeply. You can also contract your pelvic floor muscles with each exhale while holding bridge pose. When you lower, slowly bring your hips back to the ground articulating the spine vertebrae by vertebrae onto the ground.

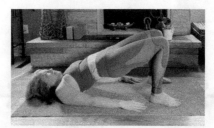

Bridge Pose

Cat and cow pose *(Bitilasana Marjaryasana)*

Cat and cow is an excellent every day warm up to increase mobility and flexibility in your spine and begin to activate those pelvic floor muscles.

Start on your hands and knees with your hands directly underneath your shoulders and your knees underneath your hips for proper alignment.

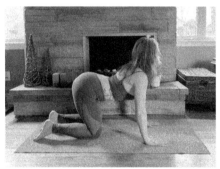

Inhale in cat pose.

When you inhale, you tilt your pelvis back, arching your lower spine so your abdomen dips closer to the ground, look up, sticking your chest out.

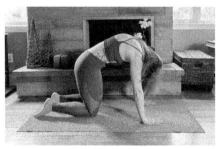

Exhale in cow pose.

When you exhale, you tilt your pelvis forward , curving your spine back and up towards the sky. Head follows the spine coming down and you can also pull in your abdominal muscles.

Continue this fluid motion with each inhale and exhale at your own pace. You can practice this for 1 -3 minutes.

Use your breath to power you through it.

Cobra pose *(Bhujangasana)*

Cobra opens the chest and strengthens the **core** body. Don't do cobra if you are pregnant or have had recent abdominal surgery.

Start by lying flat on your belly on the floor. Bring your hands flat and underneath your shoulders.

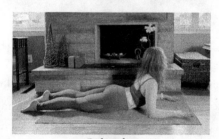

Baby cobra

On the inhale, look up, arch your upper spine and lead with your chest. You can stay here in baby cobra and keep your forearms on the ground or you can come all the way up to your hands.

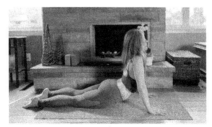

Cobra

A few key points:

- Keep your neck in line with your spine, keep your gaze down. Be careful not to over extend your neck.

- Chest pushes up and forward. Shoulder blades are drawn back and down.

- Keep elbows tucked in close to your body.

- Your hips, belly, pelvis, and fronts of your thighs are making contact with the ground.

- Feet can be hip width apart with tops of feet on the ground.

- Be mindful not to clench your bum.

Crocodile pose *(Makarasana)*

This is a great way to relax and release pain and stress. It is a perfect way to end your yoga practice. This is a **grounding** pose.

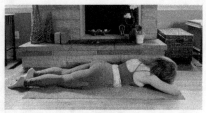

Crocodile

Lower your body to the ground, laying on your belly. You are lying facing down with your elbows tucked in at your sides, palms facing down. Bring your hands to the front of the mat. Slowly cross your arms in front of you, creating support to rest your forehead.

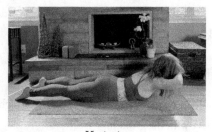

Variation

To challenge yourself and stretch your lower back, lift your upper body. This will open the chest and release tension in the shoulders and back. It will also improve flexibility in your lower back

Downward Facing Dog *(Adho Mukha Svanasana)*

Downward facing dog deeply stretches the back, opens the chest, and builds upper body strength. It also stretches the legs and **opens the hips** which help the pelvic bowl and pelvic floor muscles engage and relax.

Start on hands and knees. Spread the fingers wide apart on the mat. Press through the palms and fingers and edges of the hands. Push your hips up into the air. Keep pushing your hips further back while reaching the chest towards the thighs. Lift up through the tailbone to keep the spine straight and long. It's okay if your heels don't come all the way down to the floor. Push your shoulders back and down. This widens the chest and stretches the upper back. If your heels do not come to the floor and your hamstrings feel tight, you can alternate bending the knees here. Breathe deeply. Let your head and neck relax freely. To end, exhale and come back into a table top position on hands and knees.

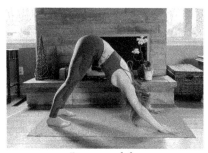

Downward dog

Frog pose with or without Kegels *(Mandukasana)*

Frog pose is a **hip opener** and relaxes the pelvic floor muscles.

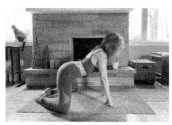

Beginning of frog's pose

For frog pose, the best starting position is on hands and knees again. Basically you are widening your knees further apart on the floor.

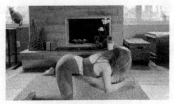

Frog's pose

This is opening the hips and stretching the inner thighs. Bring your forearms to the ground and rest there. Breathe deeply. You can engage a kegel and rhythmically contract with the exhale, release with the inhale.

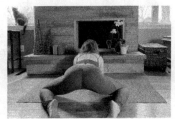

Back view of frog's pose

Check the Resources Section for a free tutorial from my YouTube Channel.

Alternatives to Frog Pose

Child's Pose *(Balasana)*

Child's pose is a **hip opener** and **grounding** pose and it is especially good for women to do every day. So much stored trauma and emotions can be released from the hips resting in child's pose if held up to 5 minutes daily. It also relaxes the pelvic floor muscles.

Sitting on your heels, spread your knees wide. It may be helpful to put a cushion under your bum or a towel under your knees for extra cushion and support.

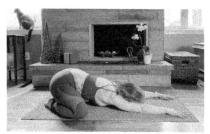

Child's pose

Walk your hands out in front of you on the floor while you bring your chest towards the floor. You will feel the stretch and opening in your hips and lower back.

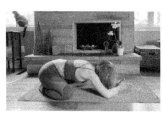

Child's pose support with block

You can rest your forehead on the floor or a block for elevation and support. Arms can be outstretched in front or alongside behind you with palms facing up. Alternatively, you can support yourself with a bolster pillow or a bed pillow underneath your torso.

Relax your pelvic floor muscles and breathe deeply. For a tutorial with props and variations, head to Resources for video support.

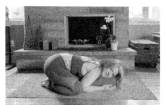

Supported Child's pose with bolster

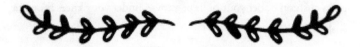

Happy Baby (Ananda Balasana)

Happy baby is a **hip opener** and relaxes the pelvic floor muscles, as well as stretches and massages the lower back.

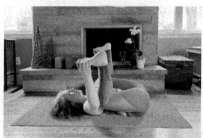

Happy baby

Lying on your back. Bring your knees up towards your chest and pointing outwards. Grab the bottoms of your feet and spread your knees apart. You can rock from side to side on your lower back. This is a calming pose and it resembles a happy baby!

Half-shoulder stand or Plow *(Halasana*)

Half shoulder stand is an **inversion**. If you are pregnant in your first trimester or menstruating, inversions are not recommended. **Plow pose is not for beginners** to yoga and should be practiced carefully. When practiced, it can relieve lower back ache and **opens the hips**.

Lie on your back with your knees bent and your feet flat on the floor. Lift up your hips similarly to bridge pose and clasp your hands together bringing your shoulder blades closer together underneath.

Then lower your hips back down and bring your legs up into the air in a half shoulder stand. You can bring your hands to the base of your spine to support. Breathe deeply and stay here for a few minutes.

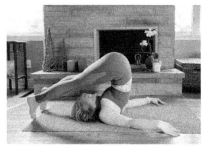

Half shoulder stand (plow)

Gentle variation for half shoulder stand

Legs-up-the-Wall (*Viparita Karani*)

This is an accessible pose that is great for the circulatory system and diverting blood flow to the pelvic bowl. This is also an excellent pose for de-stressing and dropping you into the parasympathetic nervous system to experience deep relaxation. Legs-up-the wall is a **grounding** pose.

Get comfortable with a pillow for your head or a blanket.

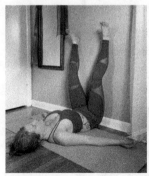

Legs-up-the-wall

A helpful way to get into the pose is to sit sideways with the wall. Bring your feet up and lay down on your back simultaneously. You want your tailbone on the floor and as close to the wall as possible, with your legs extended up and heels resting on the wall. Your spine and head are aligned on the floor and perpendicular to the wall. Keep your knees relaxed, feeling a light stretch behind your legs. Breathe deeply here. You can stay here for 5-10 minutes. Come out carefully and slowly. Take your time coming out of inversion poses. Legs up the wall is a great restorative pose to do on its own or at the end of your yoga practice in place of corpse pose.

Fish *(Matsyasana)*

Fish pose relieves tension in your neck, throat, and shoulders. It stretches and stimulates the organs of your belly and abdominals which surround your pelvic bowl. This is a **reclining backbend pose**.

Lie flat on your back.

Lying flat here, prop yourself up on to your forearms and rest on your elbows so your torso is raised and you are leaning back. Lower your shoulders and the back of your head to the floor. Bring your arms underneath your bum for support. Inhale and press elbows down, lift your chest, and rest the top of your head on the floor. You will feel this stretch and opening in your neck. Remain here for several breaths. A neck injury is contraindicated for fish pose.

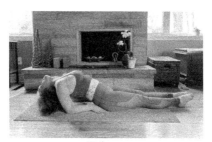

Fish pose

A variation for fish pose is to support yourself with pillows underneath your back and neck. This is a relaxing and grounding variation.

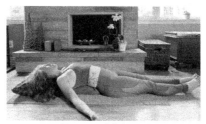

Supported fish pose

Locust Pose (*Salabhasana*)

This pose reduces stress and relieves mild depression and anxiety. It also strengthens the **core** and back. You lie on your belly with arms straight back by your side. Forehead is resting on the ground. Inhale and lift your head, chest, arms, and legs off the floor a few inches. Breathe deeply for a few deep breaths and then release. Alternatively, you can raise an alternate arm and leg leaving the other arm and leg on the floor, then switching.

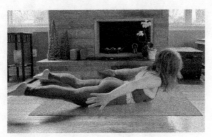

Locust pose

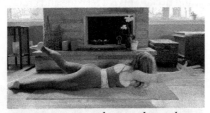

Locust variation, alternate leg and arm lift

Plank pose *(Phalakasana)*

Plank pose engages your **core** and contracts and engages your pelvic floor muscles. Start on your hands and knees. Make sure your hands are directly underneath your shoulders. Knees are aligned directly under your hips. Bring your right foot back behind you and extend your left with toes on the ground and then extend your left leg behind you. Keep your neck aligned with your spine keeping eyes down or a few inches in front on the mat.

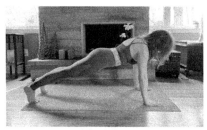

Plank pose

Engage your core muscles here keeping your entire body in a straight angle. Breathe deeply. Hold for 30 seconds and work up to 1 minute. Alternatively you can bring your forearms to the ground for forearm plank.

Do your best! If you need to lower your knees that's okay! Take a rest and go back into it when you're ready.

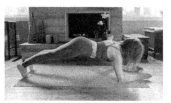

Variation: Forearm plank

Seated twists (*Ardha matsyendrasana*)

Start sitting on the floor with your knees bent and feet flat on the floor. Bring your left leg to the floor with your foot towards your groin.

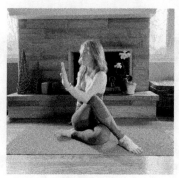

Seated twist

Bring your right foot and cross it over your left leg with foot flat on the floor. Then start lightly twisting your upper body and place your left upper arm resting on your right knee. Don't force the twist. Continue to lengthen the spine in this position breathing deeply. Then inhale and relax out of the position. Do the stretch on the other side. This increases hip and spinal flexibility.

Sitting forward bend (*paschimottanasana*)

Sit on the floor with legs extended in front of you. The key here is to leave the backs of your knees on the floor. Inhale and sit up straight, lengthening your spine. Exhale and hinge from your hips and waist forward bringing your chest closer to your knees. Lead with your heart here. Your hands can grab on to your thighs, shins, or toes depending on your flexibility. Be mindful not to curve your upper back.

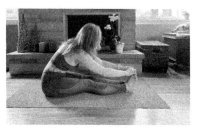

Seated forward bend.

If your knees start to come off the ground, decrease your range of motion and raise your torso up slightly. You will feel a stretch behind your legs. Keep your spine straight and breathe deeply here. Alternatively, you can use a strap around the bottoms of your feet and hold on to the straps getting the same stretch. You may be sitting upright, just slightly bent forward. This pose can help relieve menstrual discomfort and it stimulates the pelvic region, increasing circulation to the pelvic organs.

Yoga Squat (*Malasana*)

Yoga squat is a **hip opener** and relieves lower back pain. Stand with your feet about hip width apart. Inhale and lengthen up. Exhale and bend your knees and bring your bum towards the ground into a squatting position. Keep your hips off the ground. Hands can be 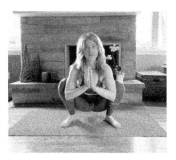 pressed together in a prayer position. Hold here and breathe deeply. Yoga squat is excellent for relaxing the pelvic floor muscles.

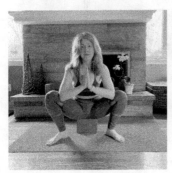

If you do not have range of motion in your knees or history of knee injury, there are variations. You can sit on a block or sit on a step in your house to elevate you. You can also put a towel under your heels for support. Yoga squat is excellent for relieving lower back pain and per-

Yoga squat supported by block

fect for pregnant women to practice.

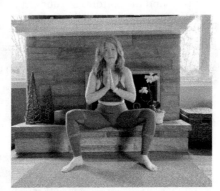

Yoga squat on step

Wind relieving pose or Knees-to-Chest *(Pawanmuktasana)*

As the same states, this pose is excellent for relaxing digestion and releasing gas which is normal and healthy. This pose will help you to relax your abdomen, hips, thighs, and buttocks. Lie on your back. Bend both knees and bring your knees towards your chest. Keep your knees and ankles together. Bring your arms around your legs and give them a hug or take hold of your elbows.

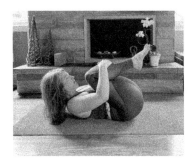

Lift up your neck and tuck your chin into your chest or bring it onto your knees. Alternatively, you can leave your head on the ground if you have neck strain and find it more comfortable. Hold this pose for up to 1 minute and breathe deeply. You can also do this pose one leg at a time. This is a **grounding** pose.

Modified Boat pose (*Paripurna Navasana*)

Boat pose strengthens the **core**, hip flexors, adductors and lower back. You begin by sitting on the floor with your legs extended in front of you. Place your hands behind you on the floor and lean back slightly. Be sure to stick out your chest. You are anchored on your tailbone and sitting bones on the ground. Exhale and raise your legs about 45 degrees off the floor. Ideally your legs are straight, but it's okay to have a bend in the knees as well.

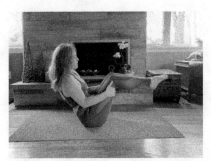

Modified boat pose

If knees are bent, keep your shins parallel to the ground. Keep your heart open and spine straight. Extend your arms straight alongside your legs and parallel to the floor This is a challenging pose. Do your best. Start with holding for 10 or 20 seconds and work up your strength to hold it for up to a minute.

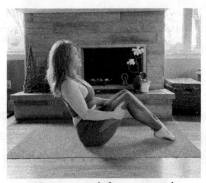

Variation with feet on ground.

Variation is to leave your feet on the ground with knees bent, but continue to pull shoulders back and stick sternum out. Keep your spine straight and engage your core.

Avoid strong core engagement like in this pose if you are pregnant (2nd or 3rd trimester) or menstruating.

Pigeon pose (*Eka Pada Rajakapotasana*)

Pigeon pose is excellent for **opening up the hip flexors** and improves circulation to the abdominal cavity, pelvis, and low back. This pose is ideal for relaxing the pelvic floor muscles.

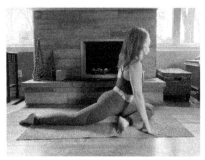

Pigeon pose

You start on your hands and knees. Bend your left knee and place your left foot near your right groin in front of you on the floor. Extend your right leg back behind you with the front of your thigh, shin and top of the foot on the floor. The key here is to be sure your hips are square to the front. It's a common mistake to lift one of the hips. Do your best! You can stay here for a few deep breaths. When you're done on the left side, switch sides and bring your right knee near your left groin to balance the other side, with your left leg extended behind. If you desire a deeper stretch in pigeon pose, you can fold forward from the waist , hinging from your hips over your front leg.

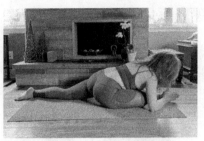

Folded over in pigeon pose

Variation to Pigeon Pose

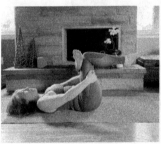

Variation for pigeon pose

Lying on your back, bend your knees with feet flat on the floor. Bring your left foot resting on your right knee. Grasp hands behind your right thigh and bring it towards your chest. Be mindful to continually push your left knee out and back. It will have a tendency to cave in. This will allow a wonderful stretch along your outer thigh and deep psoas muscle. When you're done with the left side, switch over and bring your right foot to the left knee for the other side. In each stretch, hold, and breathe deeply for 1-2 minutes.

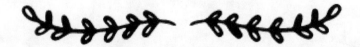

Chair pose *(Utkatasana)*

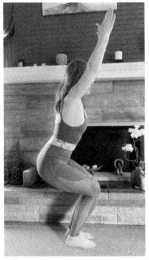

Chair pose

Begin by standing in mountain pose. Exhale and bend your knees to 90 degrees bringing your bum behind you as if sitting in a chair. Inhale and stretch your arms alongside your ears. Bring shoulders down and back with fingers straightening right up. Hold for 15 to 30 seconds while continuing to breathe deeply. To release, inhale and straighten legs and exhale lower your arms. Chair pose is a **core strengthener**.

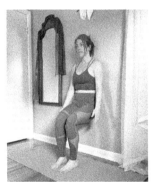

Chair supported by wall

Alternatively, you can use a wall for support and sit in chair pose against the wall with your upper back supported. Make sure feet are flat on the ground and knees are bent 90 degrees.

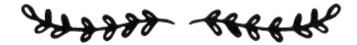

Warrior I pose *(Virabhadrasana)*

Start in mountain pose.

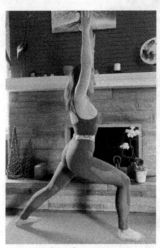

Right side Warrior I

Step your right foot forward with hands on your hips. Right foot points straight ahead and back left foot is angled slightly outward. Feel firmly rooted and engage your leg muscles. Exhale and bend your right knee to 90 degrees. Be sure your hips are square to the front.

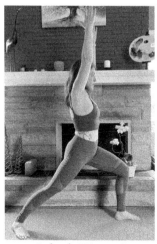

Left side Warrior I

You may need to adjust the distance between your feet so that your right shin is perpendicular to the floor and right thigh is parallel to the floor for a 90 degree angle. Inhale and extend your arms overhead. Root down in your pelvis and through your legs. Hold for a few breaths and then inhale and release.

Repeat on the other side. Warrior pose is a **standing and grounding pose.**

Triangle Pose *(Utthita Trikonasana)*

It is simple to go into triangle pose from warrior because your stance is already partly set up. From Warrior I, open up to Warrior 2 by turning your torso from the front and opening up to the side. Arms are parallel to the ground. Your back foot turns out slightly 45 degrees. Adjust your stance as needed. You may need to widen your stance.

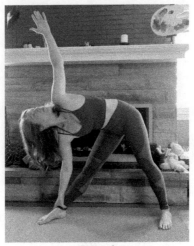

Triangle

Straighten your right leg. Then lower your right hand down onto your shin or ankle. It's more important to keep your leg straight with no bend in the knee. Use a block to maintain this integrity.

The left shoulder stacks on top of the right one as you open your chest, reaching your left fingertips toward the ceiling while keeping your left shoulder rooted in its socket. You can also keep your right hand higher on your thigh to open up your chest.

Turn your head to take your gaze up toward your left fingertips. If this is uncomfortable for your neck, it's also fine to keep the head in a more neutral position.

Soften your right knee slightly in a micro bend to prevent hyperextension. Stay for at least 5 breaths. Repeat the pose with your left leg forward.

Key alignment: Make sure your right heel is lined up with the arch of your left foot and vice versa.

Triangle pose is a **standing yoga pose** that strengthens the lower body and opens the chest and shoulders.

Reclining bound angle pose (*Supta Baddha Konasana*)

This is a **great pose to do at the end of your stretching** to relax. It improves circulation to the pelvis and reproductive organs. Have a bolster pillow or any other pillow for support. You can also use blocks for this one. Sit at the edge of the pillow and bring the soles of your feet together. Let your knees fall open to the sides.

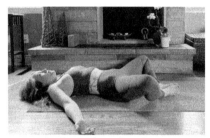

Reclining bound angle pose

You don't have to use a strap here, but you can for extra support. Wrap the strap around your lower back and over your thighs, then around the front of your thighs and feet. Slowly recline back on the pillow. Close your eyes here and breathe deeply and slowly. You can support your knees with rolled up blankets or pillows for extra support.

Goddess Pose *(Utkata Konasana)*

Start standing with your legs spread apart on the mat wider than your hips. Point your toes out slightly about 45 degrees. Bend your knees bringing your hips and bum towards the floor. Press the hips forward and press your knees back. Drop the shoulders down and back and press the chest toward the front of the room. Hands can be on hips for stabilization.

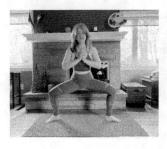

They can be pressed together in front of your chest in a prayer position. Breathe deeply and hold here for a few breaths. To release, inhale and straighten legs, exhale and lower your arms. Goddess pose directly stimulates the uro-genital area. Goddess pose is a **standing yoga pose** and very grounding.

Reclining Toe *(Supta Padangusthasana)*

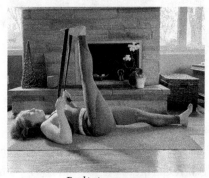

Reclining toe pose

Lie flat on your back. It's helpful to have a yoga strap for this pose but you don't need one. This stretch **opens up the hip flexors** and stretches the hamstrings. Place the strap or belt underneath your right foot. Keeping your left leg flat on the mat or bend the left knee and place your left foot flat on the mat. Grab both ends of the strap and raise your right foot towards the sky. The key here is to straighten that right leg that is extended, no bend in the knee. Adjust the strap and lower your leg to keep the integrity. If your knee is bending, decrease the range of motion. Hold here for a few deep breaths. Then repeat on the other side.

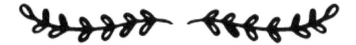

Kundalini Yoga Exercises for the Pelvic Floor

Spinal flex

Spinal Flex is a common warm-up exercise in Kundalini yoga because it increases flexibility of the spine, opens up the chest and shoulders, and circulates the kundalini energy along the spine and the 7 main chakras.

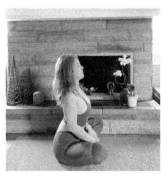

It also stimulates and grounds the pelvic floor muscles. Sit in an easy pose, cross legged position. Hands come to the shins. Inhale, arch your spine forward and stick your chest out.

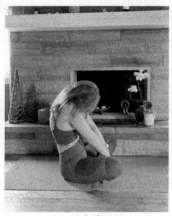

Exhale

Exhale and curve your spine back by coming concave. Continue breathing powerfully with the motion.

Alternatively you can sit in a sturdy chair as straight as possible. Feet are flat on the floor, legs uncrossed and open. Hands resting on your knees. Inhale and arch your spine forward, stick chest out. Exhale, curve spine back and contract your pelvic floor muscles. Eyes can be closed and focused on the brow point, which is in-between your eyebrows and a bit above.

Sufi grinds

Sit cross-legged on the floor or sitting upright in a chair. Hands are resting on knees in either position.

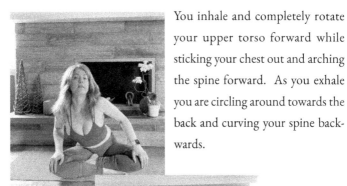

You inhale and completely rotate your upper torso forward while sticking your chest out and arching the spine forward. As you exhale you are circling around towards the back and curving your spine backwards.

Inhale forward.

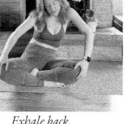

Exhale back.

You continue in this circular motion in this direction. After 10 in one direction, you can switch and circle in the other direction. Additionally, you are grounding down through your pelvis. Imagine your upper body above your pelvis is the pestle and the ground is the mortar. You are grinding down like mortar and pestle grinding spices.

I teach this as a warm up exercise in all of my classes and private clients because it's accessible and feels so good. It's like a massage for your internal organs.

Standing pelvic tilts

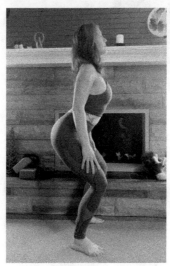

Inhale forward.

Pelvic tilts are like a standing cat and cow. You start standing with your feet hip width apart, knees slightly bent. Hands on your knees.

Inhale and arch your spine forward while you stick your chest out and shoulders back. Look up.

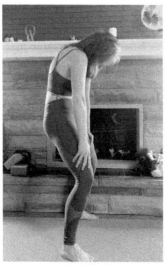

Exhale back.

Exhale and curve your spine back. Contract your pelvic floor muscles and core on the exhale. Repeat rhythmically with your breath.

Sat Kriya

The word kriya means "action." In kundalini yoga, a kriya is an exercise or a specific sequence of exercises that works towards an outcome. Sat Kriya is a single exercise that is excellent to practice every day for 3 minutes. It strengthens the entire sexual system and physically the internal organs receive a gentle massage. Beginner's should start with 1 minute.

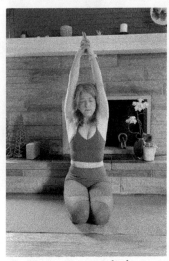

*Sat Kriya, sitting on heels, inter-
lace fingers.*

You sit on your heels. Interlace your fingers and point index fingers
straight up.

There is a mantra that is used *"**Sat Nam.**"* Sat Nam means "I am
truth." With the "Sat" you pull in your navel point and contract your
pelvic floor muscles. With "Nam" you relax the belly and the pelvic
floor muscles. You repeat this contraction and release with each "Sat"
and "Nam" for 1-3 minutes.

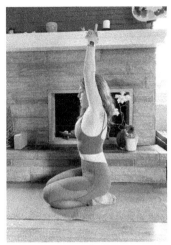

Sat Kriya, side alignment

At the end of the practice, you inhale and imagine drawing up the energy from the base of your spine and contract your pelvic floor muscles. Then, exhale and release the pelvic floor muscle contraction. Repeat this 2 more times keeping your arms up. At the end, exhale and lower your arms slowly. Ideally, you should relax for the same amount of time you practiced or double time. Relax in corpse pose or legs-up-the-wall.

Chapter Eight

Carving Out a Regular Practice

Benefits of pelvic floor yoga

Yoga is extremely beneficial to health and well-being, and practicing yoga specifically for your pelvic floor is a great way to bring more health and vitality to the area. Pelvic yoga is a reliable and effective method for boosting your pelvic floor health, lowering the probability of discomfort and problems, and improving general physical and sexual fitness. It's a subset of yoga that builds and tones the pelvic muscles.

There are many types of yoga poses for the pelvic floor, and each can help strengthen, heal, energize, relax, restore, and harmonize the pelvic floor muscles. Poses such as the Wide-Legged Squat provide a deep stretch and release for the pelvic floor muscles. The frog pose, fish pose, locust pose, plank pose, sitting forward bend, and seated twist may be beneficial for urinary incontinence (Pang et al., 2017). Other poses, such as the Bound Angle Pose, help open your pelvis by increasing the external rotation of your hips and promoting hip and hamstring flexibility. Like all yoga movements, poses for the pelvic floor can help you connect your mind and body for increased self-awareness. A pelvic floor yoga practice helps create more balance within your pelvic floor and throughout your whole body. A regular pelvic floor yoga practice can help you connect with your body more deeply. You will feel great on the yoga mat and in your everyday life.

Strengthening the pelvic region, including the muscles of the urethra, vagina, and anus, improves pelvic health in general. It prevents or improves urinary or bowel incontinence conditions and enhances sexual satisfaction. In addition, daily practice will encourage the health of the entire reproductive system; help prevent a prolapsed uterus or prolapsed bladder; reduce the risk of hemorrhoids, especially during pregnancy and childbirth; and, for pregnant women, help prevent tears in the perineum during delivery. Pelvic floor exercises aid in postpartum recovery. Pelvic floor exercises also ease the transition into menopause and maintain female health into older age.

Different yoga postures can increase patients' muscle awareness and help in learning to correct themselves. Pelvic floor yoga exercises are tailored to help maintain the balance of the vital muscles that affect the anatomy of the lower back and pelvis (Ripoll & Mahowald, 2002).

Yoga can be used as an alternative treatment strategy for women who do not have access to specialists or choose not to use pharmacological or surgical therapy.

Pelvic floor yoga can be your primary form of pelvic floor muscle exercise, or you can incorporate other types of exercise you may already be doing. For instance, if you would like to incorporate the Kegel exercises described earlier, you can do so before or after your pelvic floor yoga practice, do them on the days you do not practice pelvic floor yoga, or add them to your yoga practice. Do whatever feels most comfortable.

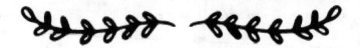

Making pelvic floor yoga a habit

It should go without saying that frequent and consistent yoga practice is essential if you want to experience benefits and improvements in your pelvic floor muscles and general health. You will eventually witness the outcomes you have outlined as your objectives. To enjoy the process and get the outcomes you want, you must be kind and patient with yourself.

You don't have to practice yoga for hours every day to see the kind of results you want. Just make sure you practice regularly and consistently. Simply spend 10 minutes practicing a few short pelvic floor yoga sequences every other day. If you have longer available time but only once or twice a week, consider practicing for one hour once a week and shorter durations on the other days. These are just examples—customize your practice to fit your schedule and lifestyle. Your practice doesn't have to be on the same day or at the same times every week—as long as you practice, you will see results.

Things to know about yoga

This section covers the basic things you need to practice pelvic floor yoga at home or wherever you want.

- **Find a safe space**

You can practice anywhere you like, your home, office, outdoors, or anywhere you need to, as long as you feel comfortable and have some room to move your body without obstructions. The space should be big enough to fit a yoga mat with several feet around the mat to move your arms and legs. It should also be on level ground, so you can balance without falling over. This practice space should be a somewhat quiet place so you can focus on what you are doing. If you have others in the house with you, you may want to use earplugs or wireless headphones with soft, calming music to prevent distractions from outside noise.

- **Choosing the right clothes**

While practicing pelvic yoga, it is important to dress for the experience. Clothes are an important aspect of our lives. The right clothes make us feel in charge. Your clothes should always compliment your activities. When choosing your yoga outfit, always wear comfortable and slightly loose ones. Since yoga involves many bending and stretching moves, wearing loose-fitting outfits will allow all your joints, and thus your entire body, to move freely and easily. Trust me, this is very handy. If your clothing is too tight or restrictive, you may not be able to move freely enough to execute the yoga poses. Wearing loose-fitting, breathable clothes will ensure proper air circulation throughout the body while working out.

Since yoga also involves bending postures, ensure that your garments are tight enough not to slide down when you bend over.

Finally, if you're feeling cold, put on a jumper. Just remember, the jumper should also allow free body movement. Simple. Now, on to the next tip.

- **Proper props**

You can practice yoga anywhere; you only need yourself and some space to move. However, certain props can make your yoga experience more comfortable and accessible.

Here are some props you may find useful:

- Bolster

- Strap

- Yoga blanket

- Yoga blocks (foam, cork, or wooden)

- Yoga mat

The most important prop you'll need from this list is a yoga mat because other alternatives, such as blankets or towels, do not provide the traction required to remain stable in some poses. However, you can substitute household items for the other props if needed. The blocks can be substituted with thick books, and the blanket can be replaced with a regular blanket or thick towels. Use a sturdy scarf or belt for the strap, and for the bolster, use bed pillows.

- **Practice, practice, practice!**

It takes time to make strides at something. The same applies to yoga. It is totally possible to develop your own yoga practice. You don't even have to leave your house. I find my practice is more achievable when it's 30 minutes, but I encourage my clients that 5-10 minutes of pelvic floor yoga every day is better than nothing at all. The transformation you can experience with 5-10 minutes a day is huge!

My own client shared her experience after only 3 virtual sessions with me.

I loved working with Heather. I began working with her for pelvic floor issues. At the age of 54, I was having major troubles with peeing my pants. I was always aware of how full my bladder was at any given point and I dared not laugh if a bathroom was not near. Any time I sneezed, I did so running to the bathroom. I also would have leakage if I picked up anything heavy. It was quite pervasive to the point where I would restrict my liquids in many situations. Right away, I felt an incredible difference. Heather shared exercises that were easy and very effective. Also, they were exercises that I could do anywhere. Driving in my car, while making dinner, doing housework, while working on the computer, etc. By the time we had our third session, my life had radically changed. I was even able to sneeze and not have my bladder release! This is life changing for me and I am so grateful.

It's worth repeating that you need to practice yoga regularly and consistently to see results and improvements in your pelvic floor muscles and overall health. It's always a good idea to get instruction from an experienced yoga instructor for focused attention. Over time, you will see the results you have set as your goals. Being kind, gentle, and patient with yourself is key to enjoying the process and achieving positive results.

It's also important to set goals for yourself. What goal do I have for my pelvic floor yoga practice? Set small and measurable goals for yourself that you can work toward. Smaller goals are more helpful because they're easier to reach, and once you reach them, you build your self-confidence to achieve the next goal.

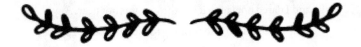

Yoga breathing

For pelvic floor yoga practice and yoga in general, the importance of the breath, or prana, cannot be overstated. When practicing yoga, it's critical to know how to breathe properly to maintain the health of your pelvic floor muscles. It is also good to know how to coordinate your movement in yoga with your inhales and exhales. When you practice yoga, knowing how to breathe through your body properly will make you feel more energized, healthy, peaceful, and rejuvenated.

The life force and your source of strength and energy are called prana in yoga. Prana, when practiced correctly, can improve how your entire body feels, including your pelvic floor. When doing pelvic floor yoga, you'll pay close attention to breathing through the pelvis and lower abdominals. You can achieve this by picturing and sensing your abdominals and pelvic floor opening up and letting air in as you inhale. When you exhale, the pelvic floor muscles lift, and the abdominal muscles contract back inward to softly and gradually remove the air from your body.

Yoga pushes you to breathe in and out via your nose, not your mouth. There are several advantages to breathing through your nose, but the primary one is that it filters the air more effectively than doing so via your mouth.

Connect to your pelvic floor

The following exercise will allow you to practice feeling the connection between your breath, pelvic floor, and abdominal muscles. The more you practice, the better you maintain this connection throughout your yoga practice.

- Lie on your back, feet flat on the ground keeping your knees bent.

- Place a yoga block (or book or pillow) between your knees, keeping thighs hip-width apart and parallel. Ensure a gap between your lower back and the ground for a neutral spine position.

- Close your eyes and breathe deeply in and out through your nose. Feel the pelvic floor and lower abdominals expand as you inhale, and feel them contract as you exhale. Repeat for

8 to 10 full breaths.

Examples of Sequences

10- 15 minute practice

Start with Womb Breathing 1 minute

Spinal flex 1minute

Cat & Cow 1 minute

Downward Dog 1 minute

Plank 1 minute

Cobra 1 minute

Child's pose 1 minute

Bridge pose with hip circles 1 minute

Legs-up-the-wall 1 minute or longer

When you have more time, lengthen the time you hold the poses and add in different poses to practice. For example, in the above sequence you may add in more standing poses such as Warrior and Triangle. Alternatively, on the days you have 5 minutes, warm up with some breathing. Do a set of 10 kegels and choose one posture to practice. Yoga is about flexibility – body and mind. Practicing for 5 minutes every day will make a huge difference overall. The small habits compound to create incredible change.

Track your progress

As your yoga practice develops, you will start seeing beneficial changes in your pelvic floor and body. You can start to experience stronger or less pelvic pain. You also may notice some of your related symptoms start to heal and slowly improve. It all depends on the stage you are practicing pelvic floor yoga and your unique situation. You'll experience pelvic floor exercises extremely differently if you're pregnant and trying to speed up labor than recovering from surgery there. For each person, progress and improvement will take different forms.

You may want to set goals and check in with yourself to ensure you are progressing. Different ways to measure progress include assessing for more energy, less incontinence, increased core muscle strength, less pain, improved muscle flexibility, improved joint mobility, more confidence, improved self-esteem, and more. If your goal is to feel less pain and experience less incontinence throughout the day, after a week or two of regular practice, check in with yourself to evaluate any improvements in those areas. If you're not experiencing the desired progress, perhaps tweaking your yoga practice slightly will allow you to achieve your goals more efficiently.

Consistency is key in yoga practice, so keep that in mind. Regular practice is the only way you will make real progress. You are not required to practice daily as a result. It just entails constant and regular practice. Depending on your schedule and comfort level, you might practice for an hour once a week or 10 to 15 minutes every other day. After keeping up a practice for a few weeks or months, you might see minor advancements. If you don't notice changes in the time you had anticipated, try not to get discouraged. If you are kind to yourself and patient with yourself, you will undoubtedly see the changes you want in a suitable timeframe.

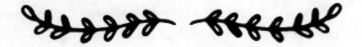

Conclusion

I'll tell you this, your pelvic floor and all its surrounding muscles are to your body what a structural frame is to a building; foundational. The pelvic floor muscles extend from hip to hip and back to front. They also support the reproductive and excretory organs, including the uterus, rectum, and bowels, as described in Chapter 4. As part of your core, the pelvic floor muscles support overall balance, sexual arousal, orgasms, and the spine. But just like all other muscles, the pelvic floor muscles can weaken due to disuse, childbirth, pregnancy, age, menopause, obesity, chronic constipation, and improper form during weightlifting. The main subject of this book is rehabilitation at any stage, a very critical topic in women's health.

Pelvic floor rehabilitation through yoga has been proven to speed up the recovery of the pelvic floor muscles, particularly tension, and elasticity. It also has an excellent effect on preventing and treating postpartum relaxation and prolapse, incontinence, and other disorders of the pelvic floor. The same stress-relief benefits yoga brings to your thoughts help with pelvic floor tension. Stress is a well-documented cause of tension build-up in muscle groups.

The benefits of pelvic yoga and other targeted exercises on the pelvic floor are endless, really. But we must first learn to speak up about these issues if we want to enjoy those benefits. The truth is pelvic floor dysfunction is treatable and manageable, but we must start by shedding a spotlight on the pelvic floor and pelvic floor dysfunction. Awareness is critical; that's where it all starts. The conversation has started, and many women are just starting to realize the importance of pelvic floor health. Still, this isn't enough; more needs to be done – so much more.

The lack of information and support around these issues is alarming, and it's impacting the sexual, professional, and social lives of many women. Chapters 2 and 3 are deep, analyzing why pelvic floor dysfunction is stigmatized and continues to be shrouded in a dark veil of silence and discomfort. The silence increases the chances that women suffer without knowing that effective treatment alternatives are available for many pelvic floor issues. We must start by breaking down the stigmas surrounding pelvic health and searching for treatment if we are genuinely interested in promoting women's health and wellness. It's time we started discussing these issues openly and seeking help from people specializing in pelvic floor and the issues surrounding it. And no, we can't sit around waiting for someone to do this for us – we have to go out and be our own advocates, and we should start by educating ourselves.

You don't have to feel embarrassed about your pelvic floor issues or ashamed when discussing sex and sexuality. Pelvic floor professionals are well-trained to give you safe and effective treatment options to help improve discomfort and painful sex, bowel movements, and urination. When we break down pelvic health stigma and educate ourselves on available treatment options, we'll encourage more women to seek help and support without fear, shame, or judgment. We are all worthy and deserve access to quality healthcare that helps us with our unique symptoms and specific concerns.

Goddesses, let's start the conversation, educate others, share everything we know with each other, and empower one another with critical knowledge about this fundamental aspect of womanhood. Let's not let stigma hold us back – let's take charge of our pelvic health; let's start right now.

About Author

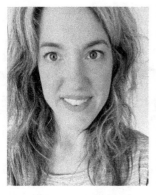 Heather was a nurse for 14 years and always had a passion for holistic health, bringing presence and the whole person into her nursing practice. Her passion in nursing truly was connecting to humans, hearing their stories, and offering healing and support. Heather has been a yoga practitioner and instructor for even longer, completing her yoga teacher training in 2006 in Kundalini yoga and Hatha yoga. Her unique medical background blends beautifully with her experience with yoga and bringing the importance of pelvic floor yoga roots in this book.

Underlying all of her work, is her mission to live 'outside of the box', show others it's possible, and raise awareness of the taboos and shame that exists in our society. She loves to dance and sing, spend time with her kids and pets, and explore her own healing with plant medicine. Heather is passionate about giving permission to men and women to release shame, bypass anxiety, be moved to make waves, come home to stillness, and BE RADIANT.

Resources

FREE Pelvic Freedom 3-day mini-video series

https://www.heatheronhealth.com/pages/pelvicfreedom

Pelvic Floor Yoga Series www.heatheronhealth.com

YouTube Channel – Yoga Tutorials

https://youtube.com/@consciouswomanheatherdolson

References

Abrams, P., Cardozo, L., Fall, M., Griffiths, D., Rosier, P., Ulmsten, U., Van Kerrebroeck, P., Victor, A., & Wein, A. (2002). *The standardization of terminology of lower urinary tract function: Report from the standardization sub-committee of the international continence society. Neurourology and Urodynamics*, 21(2), 167–178. https://doi.org/10.1002/nau.10052

Anca, R., Lee, A., Giramma, T., & Sayer, A. (2023, April 3). *Sexual health benefits of yoga for women. What Can Yoga Do for Your Sexual Health?* https://getmegiddy.com/yoga-sex-health-benefits

Aslan, E. (2008, February). *Bladder training and Kegel exercises for women with urinary complaints* ... Research Gate. https://www.researchgate.net/profile/Nezihe-Kizilkaya-Beji/publication/5369080_Bladder_Training_and_Kegel_Exercises_for_Women_with_Urinary_Complaints_Living_in_a_Rest_Home/links/0a85e536c7cf8995f0000000/Bladder-Training-and-Kegel-Exercises-for-Women-with-Urinary-Complaints-Living-in-a-Rest-Home.pdf

Ayeleke RO, Hay-Smith EJC, Omar MI. *Pelvic floor muscle training added to another active treatment versus the same active treatment alone for urinary incontinence in women.* Cochrane Database Syst Rev. 2015;(11): CD010551. doi: 10.1002/14651858.CD010551.pub3

Bellver, J. (2000, June 8). *Effects of Prandial glycemic changes on objective fetal heart rate ...* University of Valencia, Spain. https://obgyn.onlinelibrary.wiley.com/doi/pdfdirect/10.1034/j.1600-0412.2000.079011953.x

Brant, A. (2023, April 7). *What can I do to alleviate feelings of sexual shame?* BetterHelp. https://www.betterhelp.com/advice/intimacy/what-can-i-do-to-alleviate-feelings-of-sexual-shame/

Brennan, D. (2021, October 15). *How yoga can reduce stress, improve depression, and Boost Mental Health.* https://www.webmd.com/balance/benefits-of-yoga-for-mental-health

Borello-France DF, Handa VL, Brown MB, et al. *Pelvic-Floor Muscle Function in Women with Pelvic Organ Prolapse.* Phys Ther. 2007;87(4):399-407. doi:10.2522/ptj.20060160

Brotto, L. (2009, September 26). *The DSM diagnostic criteria for sexual aversion disorder.* American Psychiatric Association. https://med-fom-brotto.sites.olt.ubc.ca/files/2014/12/Brotto-2010-DSM-SAD.pdf

Cacciari, L. P., Dumoulin, C., & Hay-smith, E. J. (2019). *Pelvic floor muscle training versus no treatment, or inactive control treatments for urinary incontinence in women*: A Cochrane systematic review abridged republication. Brazilian Journal of Physical Therapy, 23(2), 93– 107. https://doi.org/10.1016/j.bjpt.2019.01.002

Camara, R. (2000, June 8). *Effects of Prandial glycemic changes on objective fetal heart rate ...* University of

Valencia, Spain. https://obgyn.onlinelibrary.wiley.com/doi/pdfdirect/10.1034/j.1600-0412.2000.079011953.x

Cavkaytar S, Kokanali MK, Topcu HO, Aksakal OS, Doğanay M. *Effect of home-based Kegel exercises on quality of life in women with stress and mixed urinary incontinence.* J Obstet Gynaecol. 2015;35(4):407-410. doi:10.3109/01443615.2014.960831

Goblet, M., & Glowacz, F. (2021, June 21). *Slut shaming in adolescence: A violence against girls and its impact on their health.* https://www.mdpi.com/1660-4601/18/12/6657

Haakstad, L. A. H., Gjestvang, C., Lamerton, T., & Bo, K. (2020). *Urinary incontinence in a fitness club setting: Is it a workout problem?* International Urogynecology Journal, 31, 1795–1802. https://doi.org/10.1007/s00192-020-04253-0

Jundt, K., Peschers, U., & Kentenich, H. (2015a, August 17). *The investigation and treatment of female pelvic floor dysfunction.* Deutsches Arzteblatt international. https://www.ncbi.nlm.nih.gov/pmc/articles/PMC4570968/

Kapsalis, T. A. (2019, April 12). *Hysteria, witches, and the wandering uterus: A brief history.* Literary Hub. https://lithub.com/hysteria-witches-and-the-wandering-uterus-a-brief-history/

Kim, G. S. (2015). *Combined pelvic muscle exercise and yoga program for urinary incontinence in middle-aged women.* Japan Journal of Nursing Science. https://onlinelibrary.wiley.com/doi/pdf/10.1111/jjns.12507

Knicker, A. J. (2021, May). *Laughter yoga - A suitable training method for strengthening the pelvic ...* Research Gate.

https://www.researchgate.net/profile/Axel-Knicker/publication/351632492_Laughter_yoga_-_a_suitable_training_method_for_strengthening_the_pelvic_floor_with_a_positive_influence_on_the_psyche_during_and_after_pregnancy/links/60a26b8aa6fdcc28ad5b16b6/Laughter-yoga-a-suitable-training-method-for-strengthening-the-pelvic-floor-with-a-positive-influence-on-the-psyche-during-and-after-pregnancy.pdf

Li, Q. (2022, January 25). *The effects of yoga exercise on pelvic floor rehabilitation of postpartum women.* Journal of Healthcare Engineering. https://www.hindawi.com/journals/jhe/2022/1924232/

Mehak, L. (n.d.). *Yoga and sexual functioning*: A Review - University of British columbia. Journal of Sex & Marital Therapy. https://med-fom-brotto.sites.olt.ubc.ca/files/2014/12/Brotto-Mehak-Kit-2009.pdf

Moali, Dr. N. (2021, August 25). *Tips for women who feel disconnected from their bodies |.* Oasis2Care. https://oasis2care.com/sexuality/tips-for-women-who-feel-disconnected-from-their-bodies/

Mohktar, M. S., Ibrahim, F., Mohd Rozi, N. F., Mohd Yusof, J., Ahmad, S. A., Su Yen, K., & Omar, S. Z. (2013, December 13). *A quantitative approach to measure women's sexual function using electromyography*: A preliminary study of the Kegel exercise. Medical science monitor : international medical journal of experimental and clinical research. https://www.ncbi.nlm.nih.gov/pmc/articles/PMC3867621/

Moons, L. (2021, August 15). *Yoni yoga - yoga exercises with the yoni egg.* Lucid Moons. https://lucidmoons.com/en/journal/yoni-yoga-yoga-exercises-with-the-yoni-egg/

Momenimovahed, Z., Tiznobaik, A., Pakgohar, M., Montaz-eri, A., & Taheri, S. (2018). *Incontinence impact question-naire (IIQ-7) and urogenital distress inventory (UDI-6)*: Translation and psychometric validation of the Iranian version. Journal of Clinical and Diagnostic Research, 12(5), QC15–18. https://doi.org/10.7860/JCDR/2018/34315.11538

Natalie Gil, A. J. (2019, March 7). *We asked 3,670 women about their vaginas – here's what they told Us*. What Women Really Think About Their Vaginas – Survey. https://www.refin-ery29.com/en-gb/2019/03/226052/vagina-attitudes-survey

Nicola T. Lautenschlager, M. (2008, September 3). *Effect of physical activity on cognitive function in older adults at risk for Alzheimer's disease*. JAMA. https://jamanetwork.com/journals/jama/fullarti-cle/182502

Olsen AL, Smith VJ, Bergstrom JO, Colling JC, Clark AL. *Epidemi-ology of surgically managed pelvic organ prolapse and urinary inconti-nence*. Obstet Gynecol 1997;89:501–6. 10.1016/S0029-7844(97)00 058-6 [PubMed] [CrossRef]

Pancake, R. M. (2012, December). *Development of sexual shame* - scholarworks.csun.edu. California State University. https://scholarworks.csun.edu/bitstream/han-dle/10211.2/2784/SexShameAndpleasureFinalDec2012.pdf

Pang, R., Chang, R., Zhou, X., & Jin. C. (2017). *Complementary and alternative medicine treatment for urinary incontinence*. IntechOpen. https://www.intechopen.com/books/synopsis-in-the-manage-ment-of-urinary[1]incontinence/complementary-and-alterna-tive-medicine-treatment-for-urinary-incontinence

Physical Therapy, n2. (2019, December 27). *The Kegel myth*. Voted Best Physical Therapy Clinic in Denver, CO by Our Clients: N2 Physical Therapy. https://n2physicaltherapy.com/b/the-kegel-myth

Purba, J. (2021, April 21). *Original research effectiveness of pelvic floor muscle training*. Nurse Media Journal of Nursing. https://repository.unar.ac.id/jspui/bitstream/123456789/762/1/85-93.pdf

Reardon, S. (2023, April 13). Yoni eggs: Pros and cons. *The Vagina Whisperer*. https://thevagwhisperer.com/2021/03/24/kegel-balls/

Ripoll, E. (2002, December). H*atha yoga therapy management of Urologic Disorders* -Research Gate. https://www.researchgate.net/profile/Emilia-Ripoll/publication/10954752_Hatha_Yoga_therapy_management_of_urologic_disorders/links/587ad8ce08ae9a860fe8981c/Hatha-Yoga-therapy-management-of-urologic-disorders.pdf

Rosenberg, K. (2017, March 15). *Anatomy, development, and function of the human pelvis*. American Association for Anatomy. https://anatomypubs.onlinelibrary.wiley.com/doi/10.1002/ar.23561

Sandoiu, A. (2018, September 7). *Yoga: Benefits for sexual function*. https://www.medicalnewstoday.com/articles/323003

School, H. M. (2010, April 1). *In the journals: Yoga may help improve women's sexual function*. Harvard Health. https://www.health.harvard.edu/newsletter_article/yoga-may-help-improve-womens-sexual-function

Schupak A. *Here is the right way to do Kegel exercises.* SELF Mag. December 2015. https://www.self.com/story/here-is-the-right-way-to-do-kegel-exercises

Seladi-Schulman, J. (2018a, July 30). *Female pelvis diagram: Anatomy, function of bones, muscles, ligaments.* Healthline. https://www.healthline.com/human-body-maps/female-pelvis

Services, Scotland, N. (n.d.). Scottish Health Service Costs - Information Services Division. National Services Scotland. https://www.isdscotland.org/Health-Topics/Finance/Publications/2018-11-20/2018-11-20-Costs-Report.pdf

Sweta, K. M. (2021, August 4). *Assessment of the effect of mulabandha yoga therapy in healthy women, stigmatized for pelvic floor dysfunctions: A randomized controlled trial.* Journal of Ayurveda and Integrative Medicine. https://www.sciencedirect.com/science/article/pii/S0975947621000577

Superpower Your Kegels for a Healthy Pelvic Floor—and Better Sex. https://goop.com/wellness/sexual-health/superpower-your-kegels-for-a-healthy-pelvic-floor-and-better-sex/

Tasca, C., Rapetti, M., Carta, M. G., & Fadda, B. (2012). *Women and hysteria in the history of Mental Health.* Clinical practice and epidemiology in mental health : CP & EMH. https://www.ncbi.nlm.nih.gov/pmc/articles/PMC3480686/

Tiven, L. (2016, June 1). *7 absurd examples of* slut-shaming they don't teach you in history class. ATTN. https://archive.attn.com/stories/8671/slut-shaming-history-chart

The Mystical Qabalah - illuminatiorderoto.com (n.d.). http://illumi-natiorderoto.com/resources/Dion-Fortune-Mystical-Qabala.pdf

Vinchurkar, S. A., & Arankalle. D. V. (2015). *Integrating yoga therapy in the management of urinary incontinence: A case report.* Journal of Evidence-Based Complementary & Alternative Medicine, 20(2), 154–156. https://doi.org/10.1177/2156587214563311

Wang, Y. (2016, August 2). *Sexual objectification of women in advertising.* GRIN. https://www.grin.com/document/337767

What is the best stone for yoni eggs? The Empowered Woman. (2018). https://theempowered-woman.ca/what-is-the-best-stone-for-yoni-eggs

White, T. (2021, August 27). *How to overcome shame around sex.* Psych Central. https://psychcentral.com/health/sex-shame

World Health Organization. (1997). WHOQOL: *Measuring quality of life.* https://apps.who.int/iris/handle/10665/63482

YouTube. (2019). *Rethinking Postpartum Care.* YouTube. from https://www.youtube.com/watch?v=8Uc398hnc24.

Also By Author

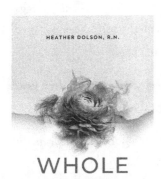

HEATHER DOLSON, R.N.

WHOLE

NAVIGATING THE TRAUMA
OF PREGNANCY LOSS

Pregnancy loss is a taboo subject with so many women and partners suffering in silence. This full-length book is a holistic navigation guide for the mother, her loved one, or partner who has experienced miscarriage, medical termination, or still birth. This book helps one understand the heavy emotions and psychological impact in the aftermath of baby loss with an emphasis on feeling whole. Get in on Amazon, Barnes & Noble, or listen on Audible.

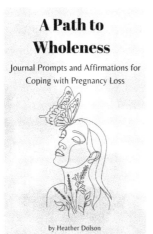

A Path to Wholeness

Journal Prompts and Affirmations for Coping with Pregnancy Loss

by Heather Dolson

This is a companion guide that provides accessible and supportive journal prompts to the person who wants to feel empowered and tap into their own inner healer. These are tools to help women and partners navigate painful emotions and provide an outlet for them.

Affirmations are broken down into easily digestible sections and intended to provide hope for the future and reprogram the mind with uplifting words and phrases. Find it on Amazon.

9 781738 838141